# IN A PLACE OF DISCONNECTION

G000149162

# Pamela Pickton

Chipmunkapublishing
the mental health publisher
empowering people

# Pamela Pickton

Published by
Chipmunkapublishing
PO Box 6872
Brentwood
Essex CM13 1ZT
United Kingdom

http://www.chipmunkapublishing.com

Copyright © Pamela Pickton 2009
Edited by Gina Thompson
Cover artwork John Holden

Chipmunkapublishing gratefully acknowledges the support of Arts Council England.

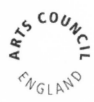

DEDICATED

To my daughter

LALAGE

Who has always talked 'stories' with me,
imaginary or real!

# Pamela Pickton

# IN A PLACE OF DISCONNECTION

CONTENTS

# Pamela Pickton

# IN A PLACE OF DISCONNECTION

**REASONS**

JANET

I don't know how it all began, when you grew away from me. We hardly meet now, and when we do you are cold. No. Not cold. You would never be that. But there is something  missing. You are not my daughter, not how you were with me before.

Take last month. I came to see you at college, and you were so changed. Even in appearance. I didn't know it was you at first when my coach pulled in to Bristol Coach Station, and I saw you waiting for me - well, saw somebody standing there, thought it was someone else and that you had not come. Had forgotten me.

Not that that would have been much of a surprise, not on the basis of the kind of letters you`ve been sending me. They are so…well; 'nothing' is the word that comes to mind. Words. Your writing no longer seems to be full of your real words  - I don't know, like 'Cheeky Charley'.  Do you remember how you always said - and wrote - ' Oops` when you`d made a mistake, a spelling error in a letter or a 'boo boo' in life. Well, there I go.

'Boo boo' was my phrase, wasn't it?  Faux  pas. You had always been such a good letter writer, your cards and notes so newsy, so bubbly. From a very early age you sent me letters: when you were staying with Granny or on a school trip.  Even little messages left around the house: 'I`ve gone to play with Jo' … 'Please remember my gym kit for tomorrow' … 'Any idea where my mascot is?'  They were fun,  decorated with  jokes  and doodles or  even pictures.

Going back to London the other day, my mouth felt dry as soon as the coach pulled away and I saw your waving figure fading further and further into the distance. I felt into my handbag where there is usually a sweet of some kind – a remnant from the days when I had to keep a small child quiet on a journey. Rooting around, as you call it, at the bottom of the bag, my hand touched something else. I felt first the coldness of my keys, and then the warmth of the mascot key ring you made for me.

Is that the trouble - that you lost your special little teddy - why I sense you are in danger? But you have a new lucky mascot now. We have one each, the same. Mine is in my hands again now, as I think of you and my fingers trace the outline of its shape. These days your letters say a lot still, yet in a sense they say nothing. You tell me of lectures and seminars, new knowledge and new clothes; a friend lending you a book or giving you some hair mousse because she had bought two for the price of one. But you never tell me how you feel, what is going on, who are your friends, whether you have lots and whether they are just companions, or if you have one real one and whether you have a boy friend. I don't know even if what you tell me is the truth, and I certainly don't think it is the whole truth…

What you never tell me is that you are happy.

Last month was like meeting a stereotype, a cardboard cut-out of a girl, when I first realised it was you, standing almost in the shadows in that bus station. You looked like a shadow yourself and, shrinking back there against the wall, you seemed covered in a kind of greyness. Who`s that, I thought, some down-and-out, until you said, 'Mum.' Yet you were once my golden girl.

And the rest of that day was brittle. The sky seemed brashly, coldly, bright and those old buildings, which I have always loved, seemed hard against its whiteness. I suggested food and you chose a pizza place where I ate, and you picked at a salad.

# IN A PLACE OF DISCONNECTION

Your clothes were dull and your faded hair seemed almost grey with a kind of lankness. And it felt as though you were acting what a daughter should be, what a university student would be thought to be like, talking of late night parties, going ice skating and all the films you had lately seen. It sounded like a list of what you thought I would expect.

'Can we see some of your friends?' I asked. I thought we might go back to your hall of residence before I left.

But you wanted to stay in the city, wanted to show me the shops, said it was too far to go. At the end of the day, it struck me that not once had we bumped into anyone who greeted you. I don`t know – should we have done?

Of one thing I am sure, though, and it is that at least one of the films you mentioned you have never seen. You spoke of it glibly, as though reading from a review. I had seen it myself and know there are funny bits in it which no journalist has covered, bits of the kind of humour peculiar to you and me. It was when we were talking about the film that the first chill ran through me.

Since that visit, the letters and phone calls have continued but always with something missing: warmth, reality, you. It wouldn't be a shock if it had always been like that, but once we were so close, involved in each other`s lives and in touch with each other's feelings. You were a busy child, full of life, and always brimming with excitement over some new hobby or new interest. You were one of those children who are always doing things with paper, whether writing or drawing or cutting or sticking. Later, you discovered Fimo and moulded the soft modelling stuff into shapes, then into objects that we baked hard in the oven.

That's how I now have my mascot, made by you. As I hold mine now I wonder if you still have yours. You made mine as a surprise for Mother`s Day, a simple little angel, and baked it unbeknown to me while staying with Granny. Then, unbeknown to you, I practised when you were at school and finally made you the same, for your birthday.

When you were twelve, your father and I divorced. He had soon realised that he did not like the responsibility and ties of marriage, which is why we had only you, and when he was forty decided he had to make a bid for freedom before it was too late. It didn't seem to upset you at the time and I admit I was a bit shocked, if also relieved, that you said nothing at all when we told you. You did not cry. You did not scream and get down on your knees and beg your father to stay, as I have known children do. No, when we told you, you just sat there quietly, your face not moving. Only now do I realise that perhaps that was denial, or a kind of numbing of feelings.

There were none of the tantrums I had been led to expect, and there was none of the punishing of me for sending Daddy away. I had been told that could happen because children often blame the parent who has them and glorify the absent one. No, in fact we were closer than ever and now you were older we went out in the evenings together, to films and concerts and plays.

*

I came to see you again last week, as you know, but what you don't know is that this time I stayed on. No, I did not go home. Somehow I managed to leave it almost too late to catch the coach. Looking at my watch as we both tried on jeans, I staged a gasp and said I had to dash. I told you not to come with me, no need for you to sprint as I was going to have to, and then have to come all the way back, we could say goodbye here. And I did run, but not onto the coach, rather into hiding inside the cavernous Ladies they have there. Then I caught a local bus, went one stop, came back, and had a drink in the station buffet. I hoped by now you were back in your hall – or wherever you get to these days.

Then I just walked, feeling  stupid and scared. I wanted to find you yet I did not want you to see me. I skirted the university buildings, traipsed up to your lodgings, then crept near all the bars and cafes, until all I needed was to find a sandwich and fall into the bed and breakfast I had booked from home.

The next morning, Sunday, I went up to your hall again, then round and round the city, the shops, the food outlets and even the ice rink. I felt almost shady, as you had looked that time in the bus station, for I was alone in a cloud of not knowing. I wanted to ask somebody, but what could I ask?

Then I saw you. Down by the Waterfront. Arm in arm. With a man.

With a man old enough to be your father.  Possibly even older. And not half as fit.

That wouldn't matter so much if you had looked happy. But you didn't, you  looked just  as you had seemed that time when I thought you were a down-and-out.

Now, you used to have a best friend, do you remember? Estelle. Two sparkly girls, Estelle and you, my Gemma. You were best friends from first going to school, and I always wondered why it had all fizzled out. At the time I put it down to your both going to different senior schools but the other day I went to see her Mum - Sylvia and I have always kept in touch  - and she has sometimes said she thought your break with her daughter was due to the divorce. We all used to go out together remember, to the park, picnics, seaside. But there were six of us then: two girls and two sets of parents, and Sylvia has always maintained that you could not bear it anymore, could not bear being the one without a Dad, when Estelle had hers.

When I told her about what I had seen, you and the man, she said it was what she had always thought. That all these years you had secretly blamed yourself for your father's going. Thought it was your fault. Not an uncommon belief in children of break-ups.

'It was kind of punishing herself, you know,' she said to me, 'denying herself her friend.     'You are better than me, you have not driven away your Dad'.'

But how was that connected to now, I asked her. The life almost of the downtrodden, for that is how you looked. Sylvia and I both sat and  thought, and then she suddenly gave a little start.

'There was this woman I used to know. She once told me she was raped when she was fifteen. And she said that she had felt rubbished and how she figured that, the way she felt about herself, she might as well rubbish herself too. She was trash anyway. So for years she slept around, mostly with men she did not like.'

'Do you think that is what Gemma is doing?'   I asked. 'Kind of punishing herself?'

'Well, don't you? Going out with what sounds like a boring old man?  Denying herself her best friend, denying herself the close relationship with her mother?   For goodness sake, missing out on young fun. A man of that age will not have her energy, not for parties and late nights and things.'

I don't know if Sylvia's interpretation is the right one. She could be right, but I want to find out for myself and am travelling down to see you again. Will I have the courage to confront you?

# IN A PLACE OF DISCONNECTION

GEMMA

I know what  they`re all thinking, but I can`t tell them the truth.

When I first said I was seeing someone, they were not interested, just shrugged. A lot of us have found a boy friend by the second year in college.  Of course my closer friends were pleased, said they were so glad because I had looked lonely for so long. Not that everyone expects you to get into long-term relationships. A lot of the crowd just go around in a bunch of boys and girls, and there is a bit of casual sex going on. But my two best friends, Lucy and Jane, have always been seeing someone and they said they were despairing of me meeting anyone. Maybe it was because I was the odd one out; maybe I was a bit of a bore. What they said was that I seemed different, set apart and not very happy.

They never knew about Colin.

I didn't tell them much about Chris at first either, why should I?  It is none of their business. If he were part of the group it would be different. But in the end they asked me what was going on because I had often joined the foursome in the pub or going to see a film, and my constant refusals meant I had to say. Then of course they told me to bring him along as well.  I kept making excuses until I could sense they were becoming suspicious. What was I hiding, why did I not want them to meet him? Was there something I didn't want them to know?

Yes there is actually and, funny, I never wanted them to know about Colin.

So in the end I confessed that my new man is older than me. A lot older.

And of course they were excited. Soon it was common knowledge and everyone was agog. An older man. How lucky. Their comments made it clear that they expected a dashing figure full of sexual experience. Sophisticated. A man of the world. And of course with money. Well, with more money that any of their male friends.

'I remember a girl at school,' said Jane. 'She got this boyfriend. Well, she was lucky. She had a brother a lot older and he was always bringing his friends home. This man bought her jewellery and stuff, took her out to swanky restaurants. We were all so jealous. Our boy friends were still at school and could hardly afford a burger.'

They backed off then. Somehow did not expect a man they guessed to be in his forties to be going to clubs and things.

Lucy did ask me one thing.

'Some of us are worried, you know. He`s not married is he?'

'No,' I said, but the look on her face told me that she thought I was naive. How would I necessarily know if he were married or not?

No, Chris isn't married. Nor was Colin. And it isn't how they think. We`re not sleeping together, either. He doesn't have much money and we never go to posh restaurants. In fact one of our problems is where to go to be together. The other is not being seen. Not just cos he`s not particularly good looking and not at all a sophisticated man of the world. He is just a broken old man. And sad, like me.

That is our point of contact you see. We are both sad. Sad about Colin, and we don't want it all spread about

# IN A PLACE OF DISCONNECTION

any more than it is already. Chris is Colin`s Dad and we are both mourning him together.

I am wondering now why I never told my friends about Colin, when I was seeing him. When he was alive. I am kind of embarrassed now at being seen with this shabby, drab old man. Even more I want to keep secret the truth about why we are together. But I didn't know the truth about Colin while I was seeing him. So now I am asking myself why that was.

I feel guilty now, wondering if it could seem that I was a bit ashamed of him too, of him not being a college boy. But no, it was really that he did not have much of a job, and we did not have the money to keep up with my friends. They all moan about small allowances from their parents or huge bank loans, but they do not know what it is to be alone and totally reliant on your own earnings for a roof over your head and food as Colin was. What ever spare cash I had went on the two of us eating and finding somewhere to go. No way could we have joined the drinking crowd.

I don't know. Was it that? Colin did find a better job, not a lot more money and he found it boring, but OK and a start. Was I a bit ashamed of his lack of education? He was bright enough – I found him good to talk to. No, that was it: the problem was that he felt inferior, assumed I wouldn`t want my friends to know about him. And somehow I just never pushed it.

Funny, guys used to feel sorry for me, not seeing anyone and all that. They will never know what a passionate relationship we had  - what a good thing we had going for us.

But however uneducated he was, however hard up for so long and how fed up he was with his new job; I will never believe he did what they said he did.  I want to clear his name and that is what keeps his Dad and me together. We are comforting each other and we are trying to think what to do.

# IN A PLACE OF DISCONNECTION

JANET

Well, I was lucky, wasn't I? I never had to brave it out - I wonder if I ever would have done? No, it was made easy for me. I bumped into them. I went there again, stayed over again, walked about Sunday morning, turned a corner and there was Gemma, with Chris of course. A moment's silence. A stilted introduction. I suggested we go somewhere for a cup of tea. Then I heard the story.

How this man's son, Colin, had come to Bristol to get away from his home town. Had found it hard at first to get work, been lonely, met Gemma on her own in a launderette. Then had found a job in a travel agents, seemed to be doing well – until the bombshell. Chris told me how he had heard Colin had been accused of stealing from work. How he had not come up to help his son – assumed the lawyers would do that. And the next he heard was that Colin was dead.

He met Gemma at the inquest - they had found her number on Colin`s phone - and now he goes to Bristol every weekend. Well, it's mutual support I suppose. Chris said he feels closer to Colin when he is with Gemma, because she was the only one with him in his last year. He just feels so bad, that he did not come sooner. As we talked, it came out that Colin`s dad thinks he failed his son full stop. His mother, Beryl, died when the boy was small - fell off, jumped off or was pushed, from the pier in their seaside town. He has never got over the guilt of that, and he always felt inadequate in bringing up the child. Then, he came from a 'bring-em-up-tough' world himself. But he still beats himself up for not coming up the minute he heard Colin had been arrested. Then he might not be dead now.

Might not have taken drugs as the inquest said he did.

# Pamela Pickton

GEMMA

I told Mum we just don't believe it, his Dad and me, the conclusion that Colin was on drugs. What Chris calls those trumped up lies. Well, he did die; they did say it was suicide and that he was full of some drug or another, as his dad puts it. But we think, if he did overdose, it was because of the shame of being accused of something he didn't do. Still, I don't believe he was that weak. I would have helped him. Poor Chris says if only his boy had come to him.

I can't accept he would do a thing like that. I believe that someone forced him to take those drugs.

# IN A PLACE OF DISCONNECTION

JANET

Somehow I have a feeling she could be right. It just smells that way to me. Maybe it is because I saw a true story once, on the box, about a boy who died filled with drugs and his mother did not believe it. She said he had got in with the wrong set and been injected, had his drink spiked or something. She fought and fought to clear his name. It meant she had to do a lot of research, reading books on drugs and other medical books. I can`t remember all the details but medically she proved he could not have done it on his own, or that there was no sign of him ever having been a user before – or whatever it was she needed to prove.

I am going to help now that I know. I find Chris a bit pathetic. I`m so sorry for him, but why did he not keep an eye on his boy? Imagine being a young lad arriving in a place like this from Weston-Super-Mare. Un-chaperoned. Vulnerable. At least they know now the money taken from the Travel Agents was an inside job – not Colin, another new employee. Got done for something else and admitted this one. Bit late now for Chris`s boy. Wonder if the same lad forced the drugs on him – acting the mate, suggesting he drown his sorrows while waiting trial, when in fact he was making sure there would be no doubt that Colin was guilty and nobody would look any further.

Knowing now the truth about the 'old man' I had seen Gemma with, I still wanted to know about Colin. I asked her what had drawn her to him, how had they met and why had she kept him from me. She said she had always felt an outsider, ever since our divorce. Oh, she knew half of families are like that, but she just felt different, that`s all.

And yes, Sylvia was right, that was why she had drifted away from Estelle.

# Pamela Pickton

Colin? Well, he was a bit of a loner, and at first she was a bit sorry for him, felt they were both outsiders. Then she found they really hit it off and she believed he could have been bright, given a chance.

I have seen Chris and we have talked a lot too. He is a broken man and I can see that he has always carried a load of guilt about his wife. And now he has his son`s death on his shoulders too. I am haunted by a winter scene at Weston-Super Mare, and Beryl standing on that pier, then this poor man walking for evermore, heavy and a bit bent, like when I first saw him with Gemma. I wish I could help him, but funnily enough I wish someone would help me too. I am so worried about my daughter – but there is something else. There is something deep down disturbing me, and I cannot name it.

Talking to Sylvia, she just says what she always says, that I must start thinking of myself and making a new life. The life I never made after Gemma`s Dad left. Yet it was to Neil I next went. We had hardly contacted each other for years. He sent the money for 'Gem', as he calls her, and that was it. For a long time he lived too far for regular access and by the time he came back to London she had kind of lost interest. Because he had gone, because he 'was not a family man', I assumed he would not care.

No, it was more than that. Access meetings might mean him coming to pick her up. They would have done while she was younger. And the truth was I found it too painful to see him. I was still in love with him, you see. That is why I have never had another man and why I want closeness with his daughter so much. She looks just like him and I can`t let him go. That is one thing even Sylvia has never known; I have never stopped hankering for Neil. Never really given up the dream that one day he will come back to us. Grow up, really, is how I put it to myself. Only a silly young boy wants to be free, surely?

# IN A PLACE OF DISCONNECTION

I had always been given his contact details because of Gemma, but I had not seen him for a couple of years and knew nothing of his life. When I just got in touch, saying I was worried about our daughter, he arranged to meet me quickly, then to come to see her with me.

He still called me Janey as he had always done (most people call me Jan) and that gave me an inner teenage lurch the first time he said it, as he drove me down to Bristol. And a reawakening of hope. Outwardly, I replied to his saying  he was hurt at hearing from Gem so rarely, by asking why he did not make the effort himself. He just said he did not know how to approach her, after such a long time, and feared rejection.  It was at that moment I realised that in a way I had not encouraged Gemma to see him. It was almost as though I had been keeping him to myself. Or my image of him.

When we stopped at a roadside place for coffee, he began to tell me something of his private life but I stopped him. I didn't want to know.  Then I stayed away while Gemma and her Dad got together. I went to see Chris. But after Neil left, I went to her room. Taking off my coat, I dumped my purse and my keys on her table and she spotted the mascot.

'I've still got mine,' she said and went to get it.

From the moment I had come into her room, I had been almost struck dumb by the golden look on her face. All over her really.

'It wouldn't matter if we lost them now, would it?' I looked at her, holding the two little Fimo figures.

'I've only just realised,' she said. 'I know what the attraction with Colin was. He looked like Dad.'

'So do you. Your colouring, your eyes.'

# Pamela Pickton

'I can't see that. No, how I see Dad - how I saw Colin - it was more to do with the square look about the face - chin, jaw, cheekbones – I don`t know.'

'So?'
'So part of me can move on. From Colin. Don`t you see? What made his death even worse than it was? It was like losing Dad all over again. And now – well, we`ve both pledged never to drift apart again. I could move on - if only it weren't for the bloody injustice. `

*

Weeks have gone by, I have worked and worked with Gemma and Chris on trying to prove that Colin did not wilfully - knowingly - take the drugs which killed him, and that he most certainly was not a habitual user. I have spoken to Sylvia and - yes - to Neil.

I made myself talk to Neil. It was painful. Oh, we had spoken over the years, but only about our daughter`s general well being, never at a deeper level. I know now that any kind of intimacy, any kind of closeness that is always there if you've had children together, hurt too much because of the sort that was there no longer. But now I forced it. Our daughter was troubled. Forcing myself to meet Neil was a bit like the moving on Sylvia was always banging on about. Or was it something else? Am I still hankering? I sense there may be someone and that it is different.

Funnily enough, it is Chris that has made me shift. For the hardest part has been persuading Chris to let my daughter go. To let his son go.

'It is over,' I said to him. 'What good will it do your son now if you clear his name? Can you bring your wife back by dragging that guilt with you forever?'

# IN A PLACE OF DISCONNECTION

I reminded him of famous cases where people fought legal battles, sometimes for the rest of their lives. To clear someone`s name, to get justice or admission of guilt, or validation. They gave up their lives, wasted so much else that might be. And really what good did it do? Did it bring anyone back?

'Don't you see?' Chris said, 'Gemma is my last link with Colin. All his last year – it was her, with him, not me.'

Gently I am persuading him and it is not going to be easy. But it helps that I understand - understand how hard it is to leave anything  behind, whether a person, an ideal or a dream .

For I have faced at last that Neil will never come back to me.

He sees Gemma regularly – and she already has a new boyfriend. I go to see her less often now. She must have her new life and I must make mine. You see, so does Neil have a new woman and this time it is for keeps. How it hurts that he could 'grow up' for her when he never could for me.

I feel sad, but I also feel glad.

And that is what I keep telling Chris – how freeing it is to let go of a dream.

# Pamela Pickton

GOOD FAIRY, BAD FAIRY

You know how the fairies used to visit, in those fairy stories, when there was a new baby, especially a princess? All the good fairies would arrive – usually at the Christening – each bringing a special gift for the baby's life; a beautiful face, a kind heart, a sweet voice, a handsome husband, and even magical powers...

You were magic. I knew it from the moment you were born. I was barely conscious and you were too ill to cry and so I certainly had no physical sign that a baby was there. But I knew it because I felt your soul in the room. Later, I always felt your presence in the house, even if you were being quiet. Even, when you were older and I had not heard you come into the house, I could sense you, even though you were in another room and making no noise. Was it the air of contentment, I wonder, or busyness, or perhaps some special gift the fairies brought? Or was it quite simply the tangible presence of a magic person?

Not that you are a real princess. Far from it. But they still come, the fairies. Nowadays, they bring baby powder, booties and some flowers for the mother. People like to see a new baby... especially a late baby, a surprise baby. A mistake.
'She's going to be pretty...' said one neighbour.
'I bet she's going to be clever like the others...' said my best friend.
'She already looks good natured,' was my mother`s first comment.
The really special fairy sat on my bed. She knew. She knew it was not just the baby, the unexpectedness of it all. She knew there were other problems.
'You know, my sister had a late little girl like this. She became the closest to her, the greatest help. Somehow special...'

# IN A PLACE OF DISCONNECTION

And you are lovely - my company. The others grew up and were soon out with friends or away at college, or gone. Left home, married. And, well... we were a single family by then. You and I made a life together with what we had, and I can see your sweet smile look up to me as we shopped and tried to afford treats. You sang too, played the piano, and it was magic. As I heard the music coming from the other room, I thought - hands that I created are sending back to my ears this music, and it is like a gift.

As you grew our lives became busy. I managed to find some work and you had school, homework and exams. But you were always there. We discussed our day as we rushed around at breakfast, or some issue in the news. Or maybe you'd just been running or I'd been for an early swim. Sometimes we went for the early swim together. Then, you would be there in the evening with your homework, your favourite daily soap. And with your cooking. When we watched television together, I would run my hands through your lovely, silky hair.

As you became more involved with your running, your keeping fit, your diet, so you began to chose your own food and prepare it yourself. Heaped bowls of vegetables. But we still cooked and ate together, and there was still our chat, your laughter and your magic. Our conversation has always been my ideal; neither flippant and boring, nor tensely intellectual. It trickles with felicity through the serious and the fun, through the theoretic and anecdotal, to good plain gossip and good plain bitch.

When we were finally completely alone in the house, you suggested that we go out somewhere together every week, 'so that we don't grow apart like other mothers and daughters.' It was mostly to the cinema, sometimes to the theatre, for a meal or just to the shops, whether local or in town. We went to Oxford, to Brighton, to Windsor Castle. A lovely day, that last, and I forgot to take the camera, but

# Pamela Pickton

I can see the day now, beginning with us buying you bags of fruit for your picnic. You in your short beige canvas skirt and my top you had borrowed, white with lemons all over it, your soft browny hair glinting with gold dust in the sun, and your long, thin, brown legs.

I think my favourite was the performance of the Messiah. You did not know the work before, and I felt my pleasure and yours as you enjoyed what I had so long loved. And we giggled about the tall man in the row in front who was blocking our view.

Then there was the time of separation. It could not be helped. My change of work, your college, and the housing situation. We tried to work it so that we could still live together, but it just was not possible…

I had a problem: I had met somebody and it was not working out. I should not have let that blur my observation of you. But I had been single for so long and was confused, and now you were going like the others. You had problems too. Maybe we both wanted to spare each other pain. Maybe there is always that reserve between the generations when it comes to our man/woman relationships. We do not confide in mothers or daughters, but tend to turn instead to sisters and friends.

We still met though. Somehow. One of us travelling to the other's area. At weekends unless we could fit my days off around your lecture times. We would walk and shop and meet in cafes. When we had picnics, you brought your apples. I brought my sandwiches.Once it rained and we surreptitiously hid our picnic under a cafe table on our knees, while buying a token pot of tea for me, a diet Coke for you.

Sometimes we sat and ate in the rain, with our umbrellas up. As time went by it seemed you always wanted to sit

# IN A PLACE OF DISCONNECTION

and talk over some kind of meal rather than walk and look and see or even shop. So we usually met in cafes and restaurants, of course finding the cheapest places. A coffee and bun for me, diet coke for you. Tea and cake for me, diet Pepsi for you.

Your favourite was to sit for three hours over a proper meal. Maybe in one of these 'eat as much pasta as you can for three pounds` places. Those restaurants always had an 'eat as much salad as you can pile on your dish' offer as well. You always had the salad. I remember now. It did not really register properly with me at the time. Although you never had the in-betweensies that I did – the sandwich with the coffee, the biscuit with the tea, the bar of chocolate if a meal were late or missed - you liked eating and liked to see me eat too. You always wanted to know what I'd been eating those days and if I'd said I had been out with a friend for a meal, you wanted to know everything we'd had in great detail. You always ate so slowly, savouring every morsel. I think I did half notice that, though I did not take it in, did not understand its import. When we sat and talked for three hours, I got through four plates of pasta, while you made your own bowl of salad last the same length of time. With a teaspoon. To make it last.

If we could afford a good meal and it was large, you ate all yours and finished mine. Your intake seemed bottomless, yet you could deny yourself all day. Maybe it was because part of your eating pattern was sometimes to eat so much, much more than I could ever have eaten, that I never really worried about the other times. I never really understood. Hadn't heard of these sorts of problems. Was just so happy to be with you. And to be able to buy you a treat meal when you wanted one.

I enjoyed our meetings, with the conversation ranging still back and forth between the serious and the laughter. About the family, moral issues, television, famous people.

# Pamela Pickton

And about food.  But you weren't there at breakfast, or doing your homework or watching your soap.  Nor were you with me, doing your now rigorous fitness routine.

One day I looked through your music - you had not taken it with you, had nowhere to play - and tried to pick out the tune I loved you playing best of all, on the piano, with one finger. Slowly. And oh it did not sound like you at all. Even had I been able to play, I knew I would never have your - well, magic - touch.  Once, when looking through my tapes to find a blank one to record on, I discovered one I did not know existed. You must have recorded it without my knowing. Of yourself, so I could hear your sweet, fourteen year old, young voice.  Oh, what seemed like so many years ago. Your sweet voice singing.

I was always late when we met.  I don't know how or why but you were always at the place or meeting first.  Maybe I was too busy, or too tired.  Maybe it was because of my problems.  Or perhaps it was that sometimes I was unrealistic about how long a journey would take, how long a walk from the station or car park might be. Or too thoughtless, careless, about just finishing one more little job.

Oh, wait for me.

We met at stations, shops, cafes and restaurants.  When you came to my area, we met at the church gates.

Sometimes you were cross.  Sometimes you looked anxious or sad but what I saw clearly was your dear face looking expectant, waiting for your mother.  Once I nearly made it.  I was not only on time but even early.  I would be there before you.  First I could not park the car and then somebody asked me the way, needing lengthy directions.  What I can see always is me running along in my long skirts, late.  You waiting patiently at the gates, in your leggings and baggy shirts.

# IN A PLACE OF DISCONNECTION

I noticed that you were always wearing the same sort of thing. The same thing.How many times had you worn those grey leggings? They were stained. Dirty. I could no longer run my fingers through your hair.

'We don't look at clothes anymore,' I said, 'I know you can't afford any, but you don't seem to be interested anymore.'
'That's because I think I look ugly whatever I wear. I don't look in the mirror. I just see myself as fat.'
All the girls today are like that I thought. They all look like that. But a few days later I was on a bus and there were a lot of young girls. And I studied them and thought - no, they don't all look like that.

I'll get her a new hairbrush for her birthday, I thought. One of those really good ones, Maison Pearson. Expensive. But I did not see you for a long time. Because of work and exams, you said. And you were going away with college friends for the summer. It was what we had always known would happen, and why we had had these years of visits to the cinema and Windsor Castle. And meals.

In the new term, the new academic year, I hoped I would make up for our separation by never being late. By always being there first.

At least one day, I thought, as I tried to pick out that tune on your piano and listened to the old tape's fourteen-year-old voice. At least in the end, I'll be there first. In the final meeting, the last waiting.

I'll be in Heaven before you. And I'll be the one doing the waiting then.

*

## Pamela Pickton

The last time we met was six months ago. And there will be no more waiting now. Not `til the last time. I thought it would be me waiting for you, but yet again it is me that is going to be late.

There was that other fairy, you see, the bad one. The one that predicted you'd prick your finger.
'The only thing is dear, with an older mother... I mean, she doesn't look as though she is going to be strong, does she?'

So many times I have run to you, at the cafe door, the church gates, thinking... this time I'll make it. I'll be first, or certainly won't be late.
And I naturally believed that about the last meeting.

But good old Mum. Late again.

I'm afraid you have made it first like you always did.

At the church gates. Looking and waiting.

I'm coming, beautiful angel.

Wait for me.

# IN A PLACE OF DISCONNECTION

## FEAR OF FLYING

Afterwards, Delia did not know what made her get on that plane. She certainly had had her doubts. It was amazing really, looking back, that she had ever got to an airport at all, she who had not flown for so long. Was terrified of flying.

What had made her get that far she would never completely understand. But it was clearly meant to be that was all, and somehow life had set the wheels in motion. Yet she thought that delay just now had been life telling her something else. Warning her. For the flight had been cancelled many times. That had been quite cruel she thought, her being so scared.

She had got herself up and out today like a robot, and numbed herself into not thinking about where she was going. But that wait had made all the old near terror come back. The fear that had prevented her from going on an aeroplane for twenty years, when her friend Allie had died, in a plane crash. It was pressure from friends that had forced this enormous leap. For she was flying out to spy on her husband who was on a business trip. With his secretary. And him so good looking too, as they all kept reminding her, a wonder it had not happened before.

There had never been any gossip all the time the faithful Eunice had worked for the firm. Eunice never accompanied Gordon on his trips abroad anyway. But last year Eunice had retired, after forty years with them, and that was when Wanda had appeared on the scene. It was then the whispering had started. Especially when Wanda began accompanying Gordon when he had to travel. At first Delia thought that her reluctance to believe the rumours was a kind of head-in-the sand reaction, that she did not want anything to disturb her cosy life.

# Pamela Pickton

For it was a cosy life, wasn't it, and it was only in that long wait for the flight to be announced that she had ever really examined it. Maybe it had been a defence mechanism, to stop the mounting panic about getting on a plane, as the minutes ticked by, and one after another came the announcements that her flight was delayed. Maybe it was just a diversion tactic, to still the mounting terror and the wish to run away, but she found herself facing her reluctance to chase after Gordon in this way.

She just didn't want to know if he was having an affair. Wasn`t that it? Wanda had been in the company for nearly a year, and the tittle-tattle had begun early. Weren't people just assuming something, just because she was new? And young. And pretty.

Whatever was going on, if anything, nothing had touched Delia`s life, that was the point, so why should she disturb things? Was that why she had kept her head down for so long? Fear of confrontations, admissions, him possibly forced to choose between them. Leave her. She had married young. You did those days. And she wondered now whether she and Gordon had recognised something in each other. That they were – different? She had never really thought about it before.

Allie had married soon after, it was almost as if on the rebound as they say. She and Delia had always been together most of their free time, and after her marriage to Gordon, well there was not so much free time. Allie had hardly known her own husband  five minutes, it seemed, before there they were off on their honeymoon. And it was on the journey home from that holiday that the plane had crashed. Delia had always had a vague feeling she had let her friend down, but never really known why. It was just some silly, totally unreasonable, guilt thing that her friend might not have been on that flight but for her.

# IN A PLACE OF DISCONNECTION

No, she didn't want to lose Gordon. They were comfortable together. That was why she could hardly believe all this rumour. Perhaps why she had put off going for so long. Just didn't think he was like that. Or was it just with her? Gordon had had a sad childhood she knew, had lost his mum when a little boy. Sometimes she wondered if she were just a replacement for that mother. For what nobody knew was that Gordon and herself were happy most of the time just to sleep in each other's arms.

All of a sudden the flight call came. Departure was imminent and the gate number was announced. And Delia felt a rush of feeling such as she normally kept pushed away. Was she what people talked about these days: not in touch with herself? She had come here obediently to follow Gordon on his business trip, to check up on him as everyone said she should, and to board the flight she had dreaded for weeks. All through these delays she had sat here numb. When she had felt panic it was all to do with finding out about Gordon and having the truth of her marriage exposed. But now there was real fear of dying on the plane

The last call came and she was rooted to the spot. Surely all those delays were an omen? She had seconds to make up her mind. Was she actually going to board a plane, or turn back and go home? And as though her feet had gained knowledge of her inner life before her consciousness did, they began walking towards the Boarding Gate. For now she had to know and if she went home she might never learn the truth.

Delia felt like a prisoner on the way to execution, held up under his arms and half dragged by guards, as the crowd seemed to pull her along, and very soon she found herself on the aircraft. Once seated, she sat with her eyes closed for a long time and soon it was as though she were truly in the no-man's land of the flight zone: outside identity and time. The feeling was one of pure peace and she wondered if this was what it was like to meditate or, indeed, to die. Was it pre-surgery euphoria it reminded her of? No, there was something else.

Maybe this was some kind of self-hypnosis, she thought, leaving the cloud of bliss, oh too soon, as the aeroplane began to rise. She opened her eyes surprised that her feeling of being in clouds was not explained by what she could see out of the window. Between two countries, between not knowing and knowledge, what was this something else? And the answer came to her as soon as the plane became completely airborne and she looked around.

It was Allie. For there sitting beside her surely was Allie, her peace and only joy?

For a moment she really believed the girl was actually there; that she had never died, but had somehow faked her presence on the passenger list of that doomed flight. Had run away to hide - to be herself, be herself with another friend, as she had not been able to be with Delia. Neither of them was a 'one size fits all' type, not in any way; but though Delia had never hidden her fear of flying, she had hidden that other part of herself. Allie had not, or at least had not wanted to. True, she had followed her friend in marrying young but Delia had always sensed a restlessness in her; a yearning, and she had always known that, had it not been for that plane disaster, there would have been some other kind of crash. Maybe that was what had been most hard to bear, that Allie had died feeling her friend had let her down.

Delia had never known how Allie`s short marriage had been. She herself had been fortunate in being able to settle for comfort. Magically, she had met Gordon and they had both recognised in each other a need for refuge. Only now did she question that she had never tried to find out if his reasons were hers; was he hiding, was he

# IN A PLACE OF DISCONNECTION

somehow just not into it, was it something in the childhood of which he never spoke, or was it simply that nobody had ever lit his candle? Whatever, those who suspected infidelity because of his looks and frequent travels, just did not know. All he had ever wanted was that he lie beside her, where it was warm and soft and safe.

No, this girl seated beside her on the plane was not Allie. Delia opened her eyes wider and let them trace, as though she were mentally sketching for a painting, what seemed to be the familiar profile, the slim wrist and soft hand on the arm rest so near to her own. She saw however, that the woman was neither her own age nor the age Allie would have remained had she merely stepped out of time and come back as if nothing had been.

Something almost forgotten trickled over Delia like anointing oil. Had that meditation brought the enlightenment it claimed? It was as though she had been into another world and come out of it with a treasure. Oh, how she remembered those dreams, where you hold the brilliant jewel in your hand and, as you leave sleep, you believe you can bring it with you. Between two lands, two selves, she had been given the chance to revisit the dream and to bring back, or maybe stay with, her precious stone. In those timeless moments, had she contacted again her real self and knew now that self could not be left behind as in some left luggage office?

There was a moment of that special kind of recognition and they exchanged a few words. For most of the journey they were quiet; reading, drinking coffee, eating from their plastic trays. Occasionally they spoke, of past lives and of future destinations. Once they slept, and when they woke, their hands, still on the armrest, brushed lightly at fingertips.

## Pamela Pickton

What of Gordon now? He needed a mystic moment of his own. If Wanda had not provided that already, then Delia would have to give him the needful nudge. They had given each other shelter long enough.

Delia had little fear now as she began to think of the plane's landing. She had set out on this journey fearing, first death, then landing to find a truth which would have thrown her into confusion. If she feared anything now, it was that she would arrive and find that Gordon was as ever: faithful and true. But no…

She certainly had no fear of shouting from the rooftops - That at last she feared nothing at all.

# IN A PLACE OF DISCONNECTION

ROOTS

'I have no roots,' he said, 'I have nothing to show for my life.'

He swept the leaves for her, Odd Job Man, no roots.

'I am rooted here,' she said, watching his boot dig in the spade. 'That old weed won't give,' she said, 'the roots go too deep.'

His boots were crusted with mud. They look too big, she thought, her eyes following the ankle up to the thin leg. And they were split. But she could not give him clothes, Odd Job Man.

'Passing through,' he had said. 'Any work, cup of tea?'

He had cleaned the car and she told him to come back. The garden would take all week.

Could take forever.

'When is your regular chap back?' he asked.

'Oh, soon,' she said. Should she retire old Mac?

Well, tomorrow Odd Job Man could sharpen tools. Then paint the outhouse. If he were not already moving on.

'You have no roots, but do you want them?' she asked when his boots were warming beside the Aga. They took cups of cocoa together: bread, soup, and 'left over' meat pie she made specially for him. They sat in the kitchen and she heard tales of different work, different places. She watched him light his pipe. How could he want roots? He who was forever flying free?

'I like your house,' he said, 'I wish I had a house like yours.'


All that week, he tried to dig out the old weed.

'You would not like being rooted,' she said, 'like me.'

'I don't know,' he said, pulling harder at the weed.' That is the trouble, I don't know.'

The weed came out and she was surprised. The weed that had beaten her, beaten old Mac.

'It will come back,' she said. 'It will grow again. That is the trouble when something has taken a hold like that.'

# Pamela Pickton

His boots were stuck in the ground, taking root where the weed had been. He left them there, slipping his feet right out. She saw his thin legs, white, and skimpy socks.

'Your skin is white.' she said, 'for an outdoor man.'

'I am not always an outdoor man,' he said. 'I go from this to that. I told you. I have no roots.'

'Do you really want roots?' she asked, filling his plate to the brim, to the edges.

'Are you going to move on when you`ve finished the outhouse?'

He washed the paint from his hands, sat down, and looked at his food.

'Have you more work?' He asked.

'You'll be getting roots next,' she laughed.

'See,' he said next week, staking out the perimeter fence. Mac was back and she was keeping Odd Job Man out of the way.

'The boundary fence is broken,' she had told him, and now she was bringing him 'elevenses' in a hot flask.

'I'll stay awhile,' she said, sitting down in the warm sun.

'See,' he said, indicating her estate and digging into the bread and cheese,

'See, you have all this.'

'Would you like it,' she asked, 'to show? For your life?'

'That 's the thing,' he said, 'something to show. But it's responsibility you see: a tie. Upkeep, responsibility, work.'

'You work,' she said.

'But I get restless, see. I have to move on. Have to fly.'

'Now? You now?'

'No. But sometime. I have to know that sometime, anytime.'

'Just when you want to...?'

'Wouldn't you like it too?'

'To be free, like you?'

'Just to go any day. Like me.'

'I am not free,' she spoke quietly. 'I have to be here. I - still I am not free.'

# IN A PLACE OF DISCONNECTION

'I would like this house,' he said. 'I'd like to be free, yet know it was here. Wherever I go, to think of this house. And you in it.'

'We are no different, really,' she said. 'I have to be here. But I like to know that I could fly, if I wanted to, with you.'

Down in the woods next week he sawed up logs.

'More tea?' he looked up hopefully, hearing her feet crunch on leaves.

'Tea?' she said. 'You and your tea. You had some. Look, it's half full.'

'Oh,' he said, 'I forgot. I must have put it down for a minute.'

'Didn't you want it?'

'I knew it was there. It is nice to know there is always tea when you want it.'

'It's cold,' she said.

'Nearly winter,' he said, touching her thin sleeve.

'I meant the tea,' she said.

'I'm going,' he said.

'With the autumn?'

'With the leaves.'

'With the wind. Where will you go?'

'Oh, just go.'

'Will you come back?'

'My roots are not here.'

'Then make them here. You've nearly left it too late.'

'Have I?' he said, draining the tea and turning to her. 'You made me wait.'

'Take those boots off,' she said, and held his thin boys feet.

The weed came back next summer, rooted here, like her. Perhaps he would come back and pull it out again. He - she didn't even know his name. All through the winter she had wandered, all through the spring. She could have gone, he had wanted to take her. Her life, her roots, what was she doing here? Roots, surely in her genes, in the kind of life her family had always lived, expected her to live. And a tenuous stem grown from affection, custom, was now a hefty stump which would not be hacked down. All through the winter she wandered, until she found the weed growing again.

'That weed's back,' Old Mac said in the summer. 'Young feller did not get it all.'

'It's new,' she said, 'Seeds blow wild round here. Seeds fly wild and take root in the end.'

Still each day she watched the growing weed, 'til on a bleak and gusty August day, she cut it back to the ground. But how deep were the roots? Roots clinging like gnarled and clenching fists. What were they made of? Guilt? Or simply fear of change? Is something as ordinary as familiarity more binding than we think?

He would come back. He knew he could come back. She could have gone, he had wanted to take her.

'I am here, yet I do not want to be,' she told herself. 'I want to go. To fly, and yet I need to be here. I am trapped by house and garden and by duties. Or am I trapped by me? How deep go the roots of tradition? How deep go my roots of being needed, of having comforts, safety, a home?'

He came back in the autumn and, in the springtime too. Just passing through. She gave him food and work and love and he rested awhile, until he flew again. Like a homing pigeon, he folded his wings with her. And of his travels he told her, his work, places he saw, people, races, and creeds. She lived it all through him, but of real individual people he never spoke. Perhaps there were none, but surely he found other friends? Like her?

'No,' he said, 'I do not know. I must be free. I must be me. But sometimes I wake, aching in the night. Under the stars. And frightened. I have no roots. Nothing to show.'

'You have you,' she said, 'and all that you have seen. You have you to show for your life.'

# IN A PLACE OF DISCONNECTION

When he went again, she busied herself with the house, without feeling that it owned her. Were not these the very roots that he himself wanted? She saw the land now, not as a monster, but something that he loved. She looked at the outhouse, and saw him, painting there. She let her hand trail the fence he had made. When she was not busy - on duty - she wandered the house and grounds and relived his conversations. And when she fed Old Mac by the Aga, she was feeding him.

She began to love the estate, not resent it. When he had wanted her, he had wanted her roots too. He no more saw the house without her than if they took the great oak door off its hinges. He had said he wanted her to fly with him, but always there would have to be 'here'. This place with her shadow on the wall, her hands stirring food, her ghost keeping welcome at the gate.

She had felt trapped by walls and gate and being there but he had loved her in this setting. What was she to him without her offerings of work or food or love? She was there, like the house, like the weed, waiting for winds and seasons and visitations. She waited for him again, growing restless. She could find him other work; keep him out of Old Mac's way.

Guilt, affection, gratitude. Was it an old husband she was pleasing or a father? She had been loved when she was young, and this life was all she dreamed of. She dreamed her other dreams now and understood. The shoot and bloom resemble neither seed nor root. Feelings had grown from feelings, and she gave all that was required.

The weed had grown again and was flourishing.
    'It's ugly,' Old Mac said, 'But I don't know what to do. If you dig it out, there's always a bit that remains.'
    'It does no harm,' she said.
    'It's ugly, choking. Can't grow anything else...'

# Pamela Pickton

'What else would you want to grow there?' she asked. 'As if you haven't enough ground for whatever you want to grow.'

'It's out of place,' he grunted. Mac who took pride in the flowers and food he grew as if they were his own.

'It does no harm,' she repeated. Indoors now she gave him cocoa like Odd Job Man and thought of her gardener`s love of her land. Mac had no children, no family: he liked to be free too, in his way, he had told her. Yet his plants and the different requirements of the seasons called to him constantly, like wailing babies.

Mac, who cared for the garden as if he had forgotten it was not his own; putting in his own time, even on Christmas Day. Do plants belong to the man who paid gold for the land, or to the one who digs and humps and carts?

Property, who cares . . .

'It does no harm,' she said, talking again of the weed.

'It is out of place,' Mac said, 'It is not right, It should not be. When something is wrong, you have to dig it out and keep on 'til it gives up.'

'Oh, yes,' she said, 'indeed. But who can say what is wrong, what is an embarrassment, what should not be there?'

Oh, yes, indeed; if it is really out of place.

Does everything have a place, she wondered.

Is your place where you would be or where you are?

Odd Job Man came at the end of the summer again. He chose the lazy days of autumn to be just passing through. How chance and casual were his visits after all?

'Just passing by,' he said, digging a pond for her. She had always wanted a pond.

It was too warm in the kitchen and they took sandwiches down to the wood.

'Mac won't like the pond,' she said. She had always wanted it: goldfish, frogs.

# IN A PLACE OF DISCONNECTION

'Old Mac? But what would he grow in the middle of the lawn?'

'Roses I think. I think he planned more roses. Or perhaps he just liked the plain lawn, I can't remember. I asked for a pond in the beginning but he said it would be out of place.'

'But whose place is this?' He looked into her eyes. He sat down beside her. Same old boots? It could not be.

Whose place? Why yours, she thought. Yours, with me in it.

What was property and what was proper? Her husband's house or hers? Mac's vision of the garden and his right as he who nursed it? Odd Job Man's vision of the house, of her, as roots?

And her? Her vision was his.

'This house is yours,' she said, 'in a way.'

'Mine. Ours. Enough to upset Old Mac,' he said sitting up and looking at the house.

'Ours. Mine. So I give you your pond.'

'He probably won't notice,' she said.

'Not let himself, you mean?'

'As long as he keeps his dreams.'

'As long as we all do. I have to go again soon.'

'I wanted you to paint the house.'

'The white walls? All round?'

'They are yellowed, grey, crackey.'

'Old Mac?'

'Too high.'

'Next time,' he said.

It would take a long time. Next time would have to be a long time. She looked at the outer walls and wondered why she had said that. Lengthy job, long stay? Like the first time? She drifted through the grounds, unsure of herself. Was she trying to root him? His roots were not in staying, they were in freedom. If she planted him, transplanted him, would he wither? Mac did not mention the fish pond. It was as though he had not seen it. She left him to his own reality and watched her fish when he was out of sight.

'That weed's getting bigger,' he grumbled one day.

'Trim it back,' she said. 'You know by now we can't get rid of the roots.'

'I'm frightened,' he said, and she looked at him in a moment of shock. A moment of fearful tenderness, quivering like the golden movements of the fish.

'Frightened?' she said. 'Frightened.' he said, 'that it will take over. That patch where it stands. Then that side of the garden. The whole place in the end...'

She stared at his old, gnarled, face and could feel the fear. Could see the weed, bulbous, creeping and reaching across the grounds, invading the house itself in a vegetable world war end. Relentless dry bark stem, and rustling whispering menacing leaves, taking away life. Plants take air, she remembered, take oxygen in the night.

Then, 'you silly old thing,' she laughed, 'Keep chopping it back. It can`t overtake us if we keep chopping it back.'

They kept it short after that, weed with dark roots. When Odd Job man came back, he dug it out again because she told him of Mac's fears. Always the roots came back, as she always knew they would. Here was her life. She thought she was his roots. But, as well, his freedom was hers. His freedom he shared with her in the fresh air tales he told.

Mac grew older, came less often. Odd Job Man asked him to show him how to do things.

'I should stay longer,' he said, 'Now you have more need.'

He stayed longer, said he was tired and aching.

'I am still young,' he said. 'But not for all that flying.'

'What birth sign are you?' she wondered. 'What sign, under the stars? Air signs need to be rooted, yet know they can blow free.'

# IN A PLACE OF DISCONNECTION

Two weeds grew side by side now. They watched and wondered about digging them out.
Side by side they sat and watched the weed, the pond, the garden, the white house.

And still he talked of flying.
And she talked of flying with him.

# Pamela Pickton

SHE KNEW WHERE SHE BELONGED

On the morning of Rosemary's thirtieth birthday, she woke with the heaviness of the years. Yet it was not the weight of age, or the downward slope from youth, that filled her with lethargy. It was more like the exhaustion following childbirth. And that was what it was, in a way.

For the last child had gone to school. She was free. And she seemed to come to consciousness for the first time, after those twelve years of labour and lost identity. But this new consciousness brought with it a sort of restlessness. Who was she? Why was she here? And what was she supposed to be doing?

She flitted from night school to temporary jobs to choral society. She contemplated a teacher-training course. Still nowhere did she come to rest, and whether doing the housework, enjoying their full social life, or even being with her husband, there was always that same hollow empty feeling.

There was something she wanted and she did not know what it was.

Then she found it, thanks to a family holiday. A drive around the countryside on one single wet day, a short stroll to stretch the legs, and finally, a 'For Sale' board by a weed choked gate. The sign, the gate, the path, enticed her eyes to the front door, and she knew she had come home. She had saved from her various jobs. Money had never been the problem. Dick agreed to help. The place was in need of renovation and they got it for a song. A weekend cottage, she told the family, won't that be fun? And her emptiness was now filled. The cottage was near enough for her to drive down at weekends, so all the following winter she worked on the inside. It was in the spring that she discovered the garden.

# IN A PLACE OF DISCONNECTION

In the summer, everyone was pleased. It was a free holiday after all, and for as long as they liked. Friends came down for the day, for the country walks, the farm eggs. It was all a novelty. But there was no social life. The villagers eyed the cottage dwellers with suspicion, and, 'don't you know anyone?' the visitors moaned. Where were the golf and country clubs?
'Who lives next door?' they would glance at the adjoining tumble-down cottage, then look with petulant disappointment down the otherwise empty lane.

'Oh, no one much, some grumpy old man, a hermit I should think,' she would apologise, and then take them off to see the garden.

Everyone admired her garden, which had appeared like magic from the first wilderness. They wondered at her joy in it and her knowledge, since none of her town places had boasted more than paved areas and tubbed plants. And so she kept her visitors, at least for a day. They sat in the sun as if spellbound by the flowers and the lawns, which stretched almost beyond sight....

Rosemary would have stayed there the whole school holiday. Like the flowers, she was blossoming too. Fat and mousy a year ago, all her digging had brought a new slenderness.
And days spent in the garden, with the sun beating down, revived the auburn highlights of her youth.

But it could not last. Dick had to return to work after three weeks, and only came down at weekends under protest. The children were bored. There was no television. At home, there were parties they were missing, outings they could be joining. They no longer found it fun to help her in the garden. One afternoon, with the midges buzzing round their heads, the children idly kicked a ball while Rosemary mowed and raked. And all the time they were moaning about wanting to go home. She asked one of them to push the barrow of cut grass to the end of the garden and as they dragged it back unwillingly, they criticised. 'I don't know why you spend so much time on your silly flowers and things, when you've never even bothered to fill that hole in the hedge, right down at the end of the garden. And, anyway, you've wrong about that grumpy old man next door. He's quite young... I don't believe you've ever even seen him.'

The children were obviously out of love with the cottage. They would soon be finding mischief, making trouble. Dick no longer came at weekends. The school holiday would soon be over. It was not fair to keep them from their friends so long. She must take them back. And for a year at least, it would have to be weekends only. But in the winter, even those visits were threatened. Football matches and dancing classes would not be foregone. Pets could not be left in cold weather. In the village there were no discos and the shops never had the latest hit song.
Occasionally, she went alone but immediately sensed the resentment. So she tried going midweek, in secret, but was often caught by Dick coming home early or one of the children being ill. They all felt she was obsessed by the place and she knew she was being neglectful. She forgot someone's school medical. She almost forgot to organise Christmas. Most of all she sensed suspicion in Dick. What did the cottage have that she could not find here? The garden she said, the garden.

But down there again, guiltily, she knew what she really meant, what the place had that nowhere else could give her. And she knew she had to think about her marriage. She had been so young. They had been going out with a crowd who were all pairing off. Like a child, she had known so little, until she came here. In the solitude of the cottage she had grown up. And there, in the garden that reached beyond sight, she had found happiness.

# IN A PLACE OF DISCONNECTION

She sat looking at the garden now. Dick had asked her how she had learned what to do, and she had avoided his eyes, with 'oh you just pick it up.' But as she wrestled with duty today, she relived the gardening, the lessons - and the teacher. The thrill in finding so much that was new and the planting, in hope. Then, the first tentative touch, the awakening of a bud. A long frozen bud.

Her gaze wandered to the far gap in the hedge as she remembered finding the garden and its secrets. She had followed a half overgrown path through to another secret garden. Where, in the long grass, they found each other. And the sun endorsed their peace.

But she knew where she belonged. Dick had other troubles. Redundancy was in the air. They could not afford to keep the cottage. If only he could find another job, further out, perhaps they could have a garden. He was pleading with her now, she knew. And she had made her vows. Of course they must sell and move. Her only request was that they go right away, hundreds of miles away. A fresh start, she smiled at him, knowing that she could not resist the cottage if it were near.

And so Rosemary busied herself with her new life, reassuring her husband with her presence. As she concentrated on family life and began a college course, he would soon forget his fears.

She did not know of his confusion in the evenings, when she did not seem to hear him speak, and her eyes held an unseeing stare. Nor how he trembled, when he came home late some nights, and found her body in his bed. Cold as stone.

Back in the village, they missed her lithe figure and glowing hair. They feared the new owners, summer people only, would let the garden go, yet mysteriously it flourished. 'She must have tamed it for eternity,' they told one another.

Only the oldest locals whispered amongst themselves....

Of the red haired figure seen bending amongst the flowers late at night. Who flitted down the distant garden and seemed to disappear into the hedge.

A sylph-like figure, though whom you could see the trees. And whose feet did not bend the grass.

# IN A PLACE OF DISCONNECTION

ON REFLECTION

Amazing how different you can look from one moment to the next. Hazel thought, as she admired her reflection in the mirror. Who would have thought that only a couple of hours ago, in baggy trousers and shabby cardigan, she had been vacuuming floors and cleaning the cooker. Her mirror self was smiling at her now, acknowledging her efforts. She was nearly ready. Her bag had been packed and hidden in the morning. How had she managed that? Now, she had picked Simon up from school, fed him and the baby, then put her to bed. Now she had finished changing and was making up.

Hazel had chosen this day because it was Roy's late night at the office. Then, good omen, eight-year-old Emma had been invited to stay the night with a friend. It might not have been so easy to escape Emma's gaze as she left with a suitcase. Now Hazel had only to wait for her baby-sitter and Jack's car would be at the corner in an hour.

The note, of course - there was the note to Roy. Better write it quickly, get it over with. She pulled paper and pen from her dressing table drawer. How to tell him? How to lessen the pain? She didn't know. She and the mirror girl bit their pens together. She was going away, she couldn't change that. Simon came into the room as she sat staring at the mirror.

'The wheel's came off my car.'
He was at her elbow.
'Mummy put the wheel back on my car.'
Hazel nearly snapped at him to go away. She was busy. She checked herself, horrified. And the tears started to come, as she looked into his little face while she slipped the wheel on. It might be the last time she did this. No, she mustn't be silly. Of course she wouldn't be going if she really thought she was giving up the children. As

soon as Jack got a place big enough, she would claim them.

Simon was running his car up and down the floor now as she traced the mirror edge with her finger and thought of Roy. He would be so wretchedly miserable. Her mirror image was looking accusingly at her now. Was it her own guilt staring back at her or was her 'other self' furious with her for faltering?

Of course she must go. Roy would see it in the end. The marriage had never been what it should have been – it wasn't as though Jack had split them up.

And yet she felt the pangs of shame remembering that it has been Roy who had sent her to Jack in a way. Sent her to the driving school after Anna was born, insisting that with three children she needed to drive. Roy had literally driven her into the arms of the attractive instructor.

She had never known what it was to be attracted to a man before she saw Jack. Cold eyes seemed to stare back at her from the mirror as part of her remembered how she had married for all the wrong reasons. She had wanted a home, a family, like all the girls did. Roy had been the romantic one, all these years calling her cold and unnatural. Jack had aroused all the passion in her, as Roy never had. She couldn't deny herself this. What she and Jack had was so special. Her children wouldn't thank her later on, for remaining unhappy for their sakes. She only hoped Roy would find the girl he deserved, as she had found her man.

It didn't seem possible that the good-looking driving instructor should have fallen in love with her. After all, she had only just given birth to Anna, when he met her. She stood up and the mirror girl wriggled cheekily at her as she tucked in the crisp new blouse, her hands smoothing over her flat tummy. No, you would never guess she had borne three children.

Now she must finish the note. She sat down and the pink lips kissed towards her in the mirror as she thought of Jack, even now driving to meet her, to take her away. But then thoughts of running into Jack's arms just brought a sickening thud as she imagined Roy's hurt. Thoughts came flooding in. Thoughts of all he had done for her.

In the small, oval mirror she saw only herself - her most glamorous self. Not the irritable Hazel of everyday with potato-stained fingers. It was as if the mirror girl existed separately, in a world different from the real one. Behind her Simon was lying on his tummy chattering to himself and humming as he ran his car up and down. As she turned to watch him in the real room of the real world, she was struck by the pretty rosiness of it all. Roy had redecorated for her just before the last baby. He had always worked so hard, been so kind. But always there had been something missing. Confused, she turned back to her new mirror self, who seemed more beautiful than herself five, even ten years ago. So radiant she had become since falling in love. Oh, she must be doing the right thing.

The phone rang. Emma had been sick and was being brought home. And as she sat down again at the mirror, trying to reorganise the evening, Hazel was aware of something that was annoying her, jarring on her mind, something behind her, not in the mirror room. It was Simon, singing to himself as he played, 'I love you Dad, I love you Dad. Mum when is Dad coming home?' Now the baby was crying, whatever could be the matter? Hazel panicked, yet could not move from the mirror. In less than an hour Jack's car would be at the corner. The baby's cry turned to a scream and the car bringing Emma home drew up.

# Pamela Pickton

Hazel smiled at the lovely girl in the mirror. I always want to remember you like that, she thought. Then she spun quickly round from the mirror, picking up her old smock from the bedside stool and pulling it on over the too-clean blouse.

'Not now, I can't come to you now,' she was saying to Jack.
'I love you, Dad,' sang Simon as his car went up and down over the old slippers and the stray bits of Lego in the corner of the real room. And the knocker rattled.

'Perhaps in another time, in another world, my darling,' she swallowed, and then brightened. No, perhaps on another loop of time. Perhaps Jack would be at the corner in half an hour and she would be there on a different loop of time.

As she left the room to go to those who needed her, she called over her shoulder to the girl in the mirror, the beautiful one Jack loved:

'You go to him…
`I can't, but you can.'

# IN A PLACE OF DISCONNECTION

ON THE OTHER SIDE OF YOUR FACE

Hilda slumped down at the dressing table. There was only half an hour before Frank would be outside to pick her up, and already she felt tired, defeated. But she must make an effort. It was a long time since a man had asked her out and it might be the last. Mother had spoilt all her chances, wanting to keep her here. Right from the start she had driven men away, been rude to them, said they were not good enough for Hilda. She had fallen ill whenever there had been any talk of marriage plans, always pleading with Hilda to stay.

'Just for one more year. Don't worry, I don't think I'm going to be around much longer to bother you.'
Until the man grew tired and found another girl.

Then came the blackmail, 'your dear father hoped you would look after his little wifey. You don't want to be chasing around in old cars and going to noisy parties. Stay and make some nice cocoa and we'll be cosy.'

More recently it had become cruel. Whenever Hilda's restlessness became apparent, the comments had turned to her age and looks. 'You might as well accept being an old maid now. Who'd have you anyway? Big and heavy like your father, I'm afraid. He always said men like their women fragile and dainty, like me.'

Sometimes Mother resorted to pleading but at other times she was more cunning saying, 'of course you go out dear,' in a whimpering voice. Then, when Hilda returned from work all ready for her date, there would be the doctor, summoned by a neighbour.
'Can't find anything wrong with her, Miss Perkins, but you'd better stay with her tonight. You never know at her age.'

Helplessly now, she lifted her head and was shocked by the bitterness on the face in the mirror. Hard, she was looking these days, and no wonder. She stared into the mirror at the faded rosy wallpaper and the tatty nightdress poodle. The mirror had watched it all, from youth to resignation. But, no she rallied; tonight she was going out with her new boss, with Frank and who knew what might come of it? They had got on well from the start, he liked her and she just knew it.

'He's probably married.' Scream. 'He's not, he's not.'
Hilda shook herself. When had she had that argument? There had been so many scenes, and they had all merged into one. Mother's eternal nagging, cajoling, insulting - all knocking her confidence. Though she did not usually retaliate, she thought perplexed. As a rule, she shrunk, shrivelled, yielded. Yet, how strange, for the mirror face looked triumphant.
Ah, tonight, though.

'I suppose you think you're going to marry him?'
The shrill voice, a faint echo in her mind.

Funny, she had not heard from Mother this evening. She'd managed to slip straight upstairs without the usual call for a cup of tea.
'That awful woman you send in from next door. Tea like dishwater. Always give it to the cat. Why don't you stay at home with me, Hilda? Father left us comfortable.'
'Of course I want to escape from you, you old witch. Don't you know I mean to escape from you forever?'
She must have dreamt she said that, though it rang clearly in her ears.

No, she didn't hold out much hope of marriage now. She started to press in her front wave and fluff some powder on her cheeks. If she could only keep the friendship going for a year, a few months, anything. Just to have a male escort. Just one last fling before sinking into the gloom with mother. She reached out behind her to where her best dress hung, newly ironed, on the door, and began to panic when the zip would not pull up. Oh, don't let anything go wrong. Let tonight be all right Let me have just one night of wine, of candles, of romance. Just one night of civil company and conversation, anything, to get away from the dead photographs, the doilies, and the cat.

Funny, in all her years at the office, she could not remember a night when she had not been summoned as soon as the key turned in the lock. Not even for a cup of tea, a hot flannel...

'Surely you can spare me a minute of your time when I've hardly seen a soul all day?'

Perhaps her mother was asleep.

All she could remember about coming home was walking from the bus with heavy feet. And thinking she'd never be allowed out. How stupid to have left it to the last minute before mentioning the evening.

'Supposing I'm taken ill while you're out having a good time? Oh, go then, don't bother about your poor old mother. Nobody cares about you when you are old.'

Were they imagined or remembered words that mocked her now, spoiling everything with the old guilt?

Gradually her steps had quickened as she determined that for this last chance she would stick up for herself. Blinding fury flamed in her head as she thought of the wasted years, the lifetime of servility. In her mind's eye she could almost see the white fluffy hair and pink self-righteous face.

'I'm going, Mother, and I don't care what you say.'

'I'm feeling faint, I'm feeling funny, I think I'm going to die.'

'Then, die, Mother. Die.'

She felt a bit guilty now as the vision flashed before her eyes like a memory.

'Are you alright, Mother?' she called. 'I'll fetch your tea in a minute.'

# Pamela Pickton

That was it. She would take a nice cup of tea and say nothing. Mother would probably doze all evening, eat from the tray Mrs. Briggs would bring in and, before she noticed, Hilda would be back.

Excitement mounted as she sprayed on some perfume. An evening with Frank was beckoning. She felt flushed and young again. But her mirror self did not look like that. She was looking – was it evil?

'I've been through a lot these days, I must be tired, she thought as she smoothed down her hair. A generous spray with the new perfume bought today and she'd be off.

And it was as she caught sight of the malice in the mirror eyes –
that she saw the arm raised to the ear, was splashed with blood.

# IN A PLACE OF DISCONNECTION

PULL THE STRINGS AND MAKE THEM DANCE

It all comes back to me now too clearly. The picture of little May forever playing with her dolls.

Unlucky May, they say, kept indoors.

It has all been such a shock, and it is only now that I feel guilty, feel I should have known.     Why did I shrug off so many signs?    But, then she seemed harmless enough, my little niece.  Always indoors, always quiet, never getting dirty.

At first I saw a lot of her, when she was very young. You know the fascination of an only baby relative.  Before May was born, I had lost touch with my sister.  She was older than me, and had been kept at home to help.  I had been luckier.  I had been evacuated to the country during the war and for various reasons had stayed there.  Now, my life, my friends, even my whole attitude, were worlds away from my old home and my sister.

But when our parents died and my sister married, I decided it was time to pick up the threads again.  I was a career girl and sure I would never want marriage ties.  But May's birth was the next best thing and I was enticed into a pattern of regular weekend stays.  Most women like to have a little girl to dress up, so I always took her something new to wear.  And she looked so pretty in my dresses too.

A model child!  Just like a cut out picture. To think I even made some dresses for those wretched dolls too.

I suppose I hoped to be enfolded in the bosom of the family, have a part share in the domestic warmth. There was none.  In fact there was definitely something missing in that house.  For example, although always polite, May never showed me any affection.   Indeed when I once went to kiss her, she visibly flinched.  But I shrugged it off. They were just not a demonstrative family.  On the other hand, it didn't seem natural that I had never seen even her mother kiss the child.  I began to worry about May, in between visits, and in the end summoned up courage to speak.  My sister put me very sharply in my place.  She was purposely hard on the girl to prepare her for the hard world outside. There was to be no further discussion.

At first her Dad seemed soft with her. But very soon he was echoing the 'molly-coddling being bad for them` views. I think he must have loved my sister once and now all he could do was obey her.

In my view, she could neither give nor receive love!

I watched all this on my visits, as the years passed. The only time he looked happy was in the garden. He spent his Sundays there, while we sat indoors with May.

At first, May used to cry. She wanted to go out with Daddy, to dig and pour water like he did. But – she mustn't get dirty, she might catch cold, she couldn't always have her own way. How could she answer words that must have been instilled in her head before memory began? Law immovable.

Though, when she was a little older, I thought I saw a questioning shadow cross her face. But she never gave it voice. She must have learnt early the fruitlessness of arguing. She would turn from the window, already forgotten by her mother who had resumed the eternal, feverish, knitting or sewing. And all I could do was watch helplessly as she curled up in a corner, whispering to her beloved dolls.

If only I had taken more notice. At the time I minded my own business. Like when I was going to the bathroom and peeped unknown into May's bedroom. She was sitting on the floor with a doll in her arms, singing gently and stroking its hair. As I watched, she pulled the doll's arms round her neck and pressed the cold face to her cheek, whispering, 'you love me, don't you? You have to love me because I told you to, and we have to do as we are told.'

To think I was only puzzled at the time.

I suppose it was soon after this that my visits had longer gaps in between. Well, there was an atmosphere in the house I did not like and, as May lost her baby charm, so there seemed less reason to go. My own life was

# IN A PLACE OF DISCONNECTION

becoming too full. But, seeing her less often, I noticed more changes in May. As her body shot up in bursts of sudden growth, so her spirit seemed to be making a fresh fight for survival.

She wasn't going to be beaten about that garden.

It was mostly vegetables at the back; my practical sister's orders, and the flowers in the front were scarcely visible through net and velour. But May had got round her Dad. She wanted some flowers planted where she could see them. And, that weekend, I watched him like a conspirator, hiding some secret packets of seeds.

Six months later, when I steeled myself for what was now becoming a duty visit, there stood the usual vegetable patch, nothing more. Sitting looking out on the garden, my sister knew what I knew.

'Children mustn't be spoilt,' and the subject was dismissed as her needle stabbed into her sewing.

He told me later that she had torn out the seedlings, 'and quite right, of course she was right!'

But that night, May called me into her room as I was going to bed and I shuddered at her narrowing eyes that had lost their baby innocence. But at least there was enthusiasm, even if mixed with cunning, I thought, as she showed me a pathetic shoebox of soil and struggling shoots, which she kept in a cupboard.

'I put them in the window, if she goes out without me.'

Next day, I took May out for a walk, and while we were gone her mother decided to turn out for a jumble sale. She stood holding the shoebox as we walked up the path, silently crushing it into the dustbin. But the one short slap was without passion, without anger, more like a duty done. And I was reminded of it on my next visit. In a way it is the most memorable and shocking of all these events, though it actually began with a kiss. The only time I had ever seen my sister give the child any attention, I watched frightened as she bandaged May's knee with cold efficiency. Then equally coldly gave her a dry kiss. The duty kiss, the duty smack! A parent's obligation, no more…

# Pamela Pickton

But that was not the only reason I was frightened. You see, before she had come to be bandaged I had been combing my hair at the hall mirror, where the kitchen was reflected, and I had seen May in there.

Cutting her own knee with a knife.

But still I did not speak. I had no children. Perhaps all this was not so abnormal. And, away from the scene, its importance lessoned. Though I had to admit the house was too tight a community, with May locked up in her mother's power, taking sedate walks with her parents, talking to inanimate dolls. Her mother taught her, you could get away with it in those days, but surely school would be better? So I bravely suggested it next time I went, only to find they had indeed tried school but it had been a disaster. Apparently, May had tried to boss all the children, and when they wouldn't take it, she had gone berserk.

I couldn't understand it. She always seemed so meek.

And I couldn't stand by watching any longer. No wonder she couldn't mix properly after this sterile set up. My sister was unaware of any problem but this time I would not let it go. The child was too quiet. She never played with other children. Since there was no sign of a brother or a sister what were they going to do for her? She was taken off guard, unused to criticism, had to listen to me and finally, with difficulty, they had agreed to try a dog.

'Just so she can run free,' I pleaded, watching May smack a doll that had slipped out of the row on the sofa.

It was a year before I went again, though in a Christmas card I had news of the puppy's arrival. But none of the expected barking greeted me and while my sister took my coat, I went up to find May. She was on the floor with the dolls in a circle round her, while she stroked a woolly cat.

'Fido was naughty,' she told me, 'he ran too fast and I could not catch him. He would not play ball.'

I could not face asking where he was now, so I just admired the cat and the dolls as usual. And she looked content enough as she sat the cat on the shelf, put the dolls in their places, and came down with me for tea.

But she was nearly ten. I had to get her away from those dolls. So for her birthday I sent her a parcel, a puppet theatre. She must like the figures, if she loved dolls, I told myself. But at least there would be more to do. It might make her more  lively; waken something in her, why she might even make up stories for them to act. It must be a step forward. And by return of post, I received an excited letter:

'Oh auntie, it is wonderful. I can pull the strings and make them dance.'

When I next saw her, she gave me a little show, singing all the different voices herself. And I thought I had made a success. As she worked all the dolls with surprising skill, her smile was oddly bright, while they performed as though they were real. But at the end, when she let go and they flopped on the cardboard stage, clothes crumpled, heads lolling, she looked crumpled too and the room felt like a pricked balloon.

She moved heavily to the shelf for the woolly cat. And as she sat stroking it, her eyes looked out of the window and I knew she was seeing her live dog. So I wasn't really surprised when she turned to me and said,

'Why is it I can only have what I can make happen myself?'

Well, soon after that, my work took me abroad for a time and then we drifted apart because I kept putting off going. I had never liked my sister. She was a cold woman. I heard no serious news through our cousins, so hoped everything was sorting itself out. I wasn't surprised to hear they had got May married off, for I didn't see what employment she could have suited. And when I heard of the birth of two girls, I remember thinking, 'she should be happy now, she has real dolls to play with.'

However, when I retired last year, I decided to pick up the threads. So there I was once more, as if time had stood still, off to visit little girls, and with a parcel of pretty dresses.

# Pamela Pickton

It was a difficult journey.  May had married a local boy called Freddie, without prospects, and her parents had set him up in business.  She had insisted on a smallholding, in the depths of the country - and at the back of beyond, I decided, struggling with maps and winding lanes.

But I found it at last, and was struck immediately by the peace of it all and above all by the beauty of the garden. I wondered if the husband tended it, or if May were allowed out at last.

She looked very content when she opened the door, though the house was oddly quiet.  I asked about the children as she made me a cup of tea, and she said that Daisy and Rosie were in the garden.

'Well, you keep everything very nice considering you have two children,' I remarked, taking my cup.  For apart from two dolls sitting neatly on the sofa, there was no evidence of youngsters at all.  My sister had turned her daughter out well, after all, then.  True, May seemed as withdrawn as ever but then it was a lonely place.  They must be hiding in the wood which half circled the estate.

Aloud, I admired the grounds and this brought the sparkle to May's eyes as she told me all about her work in the garden.

'Plants grow for me,' she smiled, 'I know exactly what to do.  I watched Daddy for so long.  I like to feel things move beneath my touch.'

The first time I was frightened was when I asked the names the girls had given to the dolls.

'They are mine,' she grabbed them to her fiercely, 'Marigold and Ivy.'

Quiet again, she spread out their skirts on her lap.

'Aren't they pretty? You're good girls, aren't you?  They sit and watch me garden and they never get dirty, not like Rosie and Daisy.  Always making mud pies.  Always making a noise.'

# IN A PLACE OF DISCONNECTION

She was talking more to the dolls now than me. I felt out of it and decided to go out and find the children to talk to.

But as I opened the garden door, I was halted by her gentle voice with the dolls.

'Still, we planted some nice flowers for Rosie and Daisy, didn't we darlings?'

I looked unbelieving to the distant mound of flower banks, then back to where she now sat on the floor, rocking the dolls, and herself, from side to side.

'You'll find Freddie down there too.'
The childlike voice followed my weary steps.

'He wouldn't do as he was told either.'

# Pamela Pickton

BABY DOLL

I would rather have had a baby doll than a new sister.
Mum could have gone out and bought a doll but instead
she was gone ages at the hospital, getting the baby out of
her tummy – weeks and weeks. When the lady next door
had a new baby she was only away for a few days and
my auntie had hers born at home. I remember because I
heard Mum and Nan talking about it and saying it was
silly and dangerous.

Yes, I was listening. I, Jane, was always listening, you
see, because nobody talked to me. In a corner of a room,
pretending to be watching ants in the garden, at Mum's
elbow in the shops, I was always there, but it felt like I
was invisible. Behind a chair in the living room, rolling
some rags to look like a doll, trying to make a doll out of
sticks in the garden, looking at dolls in shop windows.
Mum said we couldn't afford a doll. How could we afford
a baby then?
Mum was gone ages at the hospital. Nan came to look
after me and she stayed to help Mum when she came
home. But she didn't talk to me either. I often heard her
say that children should be seen and not heard. She did
tell me that Mum was not well in the hospital and later she
told me that Mum was better but the baby was still very
small and weak. I suppose that is why Mum was always
so different with Angela.

The first time I ever saw my new sister was when Mum
came back, through the front door holding a white bundle
in her arms, and then she sat cuddling it while Nan got on
with the dinner. She didn't speak to me. Nobody
introduced me to the baby. I didn't know her name for
days, well how could I work it out from Mum calling her
'little angel'? For once, I left my corner and took my rag
doll to my sister on Mum's lap. At least the baby might
like me. And I hoped a little bit that Mum might cuddle me
too, since she seemed to have learned about cuddling in

# IN A PLACE OF DISCONNECTION

the hospital. But all that happened was that I was told to take 'that nasty dirty thing away from the baby.' New babies got germs easy. New babies were precious. Was I ever precious?

At least I'd been noticed. So I started asking for a baby of my own - a baby doll. Nobody heard me. I kept asking and nothing happened. For birthdays and Christmas I got things like a book, a comic annual, a drawing pad with crayons, an apron and essential clothes, slippers, hankies. When Angela could talk, she one day pointed to a doll in a shop and said 'me.' Soon after that, it was her birthday and her present was a small doll.

I cried and cried. In my bed alone at night. But I knew Christmas was coming and so I did ask once. I did not dare to keep asking and I did not hope. Perhaps Angela was special because she was so ill when she was born. Mum was always cuddling her, singing her songs and reading her picture books. At least now some words were directed at me because I was often asked to watch her when Mum had to go out of a room and asked to pick up the toy she had dropped out of her pram, even to play with her.

But I did get a doll at Christmas! A baby doll about the same size that Angela had been, with a bald head and eyes that closed. Angela had another doll too. She had already broken her birthday one, dragging it around by its head and chewing its feet. Mum threw that one in the dustbin but I got it out when nobody was looking. I cleaned her up, wrapped her in a cloth and tried to make her better. Then I hid her. Angela soon broke her new doll too.

She broke anything and everything, Mum and Dad said it was because she was so young – only a baby. I remember being smacked the one time I broke something by accident. Now, Angela began pestering me to let her play with my doll, and when I said no Mum said I was selfish. I didn't say that I was scared she would break my doll as she had broken hers because somehow I knew there was no point. I guess I must have been an unprepossessing child - never smiling, secretive, mean looking. Angela on the other hand was round, dimply and always smiling or laughing. Somehow she looked as if she just expected everyone to love her.

I had to share a bedroom with her, and that is where we kept most of our toys. Soon after Christmas, when we got our dolls, I started school. When I went to school each day, I put my doll in my bed and said she must be left to sleep until I got home. When I got home one day, I found her downstairs, in the grate and covered with ash.

I tried hiding my doll in a shoebox, at the back of a cupboard or under my bed. But Angela always found it. She found that poor old one too and played with it `til it was even more worn. The new doll's clothes became torn. Then I found her with her arm pulled off. At least Dad did mend it but I watched him and saw how there was a hook at the end of my doll`s arm which had to be attached to something inside with what looked like a rubber band. And after that I kept seeing the picture in my head of that hook and that elastic band, like my doll`s insides spilling out.

My friends were getting all sorts of dolls by now; softer dolls, ones with hair, and even some that made crying noises. One girl got a walking doll. Oh, how I wanted a walking doll. I ran home from school that day dreaming of a walking doll, hardly noticing that it was raining. It had been raining all day. I walked in the side gate to the kitchen door to save Mum opening the front door. And that was when I saw her; my doll, with soaking wet clothes and her poor face peeling. This time I did scream and cry at my mother and told her what Angela had done. She just stood there. Watching me screaming and crying, and saying nothing. I dried my doll as best I could and made her a little bed under my bed but I never played with her again and neither did my sister. The next day when Nan was there Mum told her how nasty I had been.

'You should let your baby sister have your doll. And you can't blame people for having accidents,' said Nan.

From then on she took and sometimes broke any toy she fancied. She wore out my pens and tore pages out of my books. But she went on being spoilt, always being called Mum's ` little angel.' I gave up, made friends at school and teachers began saying that I was very clever. `She's like her Dad,` said Nan, and then I realised. Angela was like Mum. I was different. They did not like me for being clever.

I wondered how she would get on at school. And when that happened there was no word of her being clever. It did not seem like it. She and Mum were the same and I could see she was beginning to look just like her. Mum would go in and complain if ever Angela came home and said she was told off, and she took to keeping her home for the slightest cold or cough.

Then we had another new baby, a boy, and I wondered if he would be the favourite. He was called Kingsley for a start. So they were an angel and a king, whilst I was just plain Jane. You could see he was special to Dad and Nan – a boy – but somehow he seemed too much for Mum, she was probably with him as she had been with the baby me. But she had to give him some of her time. You could see Angela did not like him. She would climb onto Mum`s lap when she had the baby and take her attention. Still, Mum did have to feed the baby, but Angela climbed on to her lap at the same time, sucking her thumb. She would push the baby and one day she pushed him onto the floor. Dad did smack her then but after Mum kissed and cuddled her and said she did not understand you have to be careful with babies. From then on Angela  would kiss the baby, tickle him, and got smiles all round, including from him. She knew how to be liked did Angela - knew where her bread was buttered. One day I watched her pinch her tiny brother and make him scream when no one was looking but I was tongue-tied. If I told on her she would say that I did it, and which of us were they going to believe?

One morning, I told Mum I would not be back 'til well after tea as I was going to a friend`s house. Playing cat's cradle was all the rage then and I had left my favourite string at home. We were let out early that day because one of the radiators was leaking and they had had to turn off the water and heating. So I told my friend I'd run home, get the string and be back at her place before her mum had got the tea on the table.

As I went round the back of the house as usual, I could see my sister through the French windows. She had stayed off school yet again. Unbelieving, I watched her hold a cushion over the baby's face and leapt through the windows to grab it from her.

'That would kill him,' I said.

'It doesn't matter, does it?' she asked. 'He bothers me. I don't like him.'

'He would be dead.'

'Does it matter?' she asked again.

Was she so thick that at six she did not know what dead meant?

'I could tell,' I said. 'I might have let you do it. They would never have thought it was me because I am at my friend`s house, remember?'

She stopped taking my things after that. Then one day she came home frightened. She said the police were after her. She had taken something from a shop and the man had seen her. He had waved his fist and said he was sending the police to her house. But she ran away because he could not leave his shop and she got lost in the crowd before anyone else caught her.

# IN A PLACE OF DISCONNECTION

'He won't remember you,' I said. 'Lots of children look the same. He won't be able to prove it was you.'

'He will, he will,' she sobbed.

'I'll tell you what,' I said. 'I`ll say you were with me, I'll say he must have made a mistake and that it was a girl who looked like you. You were with me all the time.'

'Will you do that for me?' she said

'Yes, but you'll have to do everything I tell you to do,' I replied.


So now I have my walking doll. Whenever we can, whenever we are together, walking to school and back – I make sure she goes every day now - any time we are out playing. Even out with Mum and Dad if we were careful. She would never tell on me and I give my orders quietly. First I 'wind her up' with a pretend key, then say 'march', or 'skip' or 'walk', 'turn round, up two three - up two three, left right - left right.'
Who knows what I will be able to make her do. Who knows what I will be able to make anyone do?
Faster slower, faster slower, faster, faster, faster.

********************

I didn't mind. That is what she did not know - I didn't mind. Don't mind. Should I let her know? No, that will be Angela`s little secret. I don't know when I first noticed her but I think right from the start I must have known here was another child, not a big person like Mum or Dad; someone small like me, but bigger. Better. She could do things I could not do. She could walk. She could talk. And straight away she seemed not to like me. She never smiled at me. Looking back I see now that it was simply that she never smiled at all.
Nothing I did helped. I did smile at her but I don't think she noticed. So I began taking her things. That was good. She was cross with me. That meant she was noticing me. Then I heard everyone saying she was clever. I didn't know what it meant but I felt it meant special. I also heard them say she mustn't get too big for her boots – but

that didn't stop her being clever and special. I thought I was the most special to Mummy and now I wasn't so sure and anyway, I wanted to be special to my sister. I hated her for two reasons now, she was clever and she never bothered with me. I wanted to be noticed by this special girl. I wanted to be included with her games and friends. I wanted to be in her world.

Once I was her walking doll I was happy. 'I can make you do anything I like,' she said and she did, but what she never knew was that I did not mind. In fact I welcomed it. As we grew up she took my clothes, my boyfriends. She thought I let her just because I didn't want her to tell on me – what I'd done that time. But it was more than that; I thought that if I let her have my things she would like me.

She married, I did not. She had children, I did not. I never had a job because I really was not clever. I stayed with Mum and when Dad died quite young, Mum went to work. So I minded the house and Jane`s children while she worked. One boy, two boys and then three. They are at school now so I thought I'd get some peace but then she had this other baby. A baby girl – like me.

A precious baby doll at last. I am surprised she let me mind her. I might leave her out in the rain. But I realise lately she only trusted me because I am not really a person. I am a thing - a robot baby-minder, like that robot doll she once made me into. After giving up so much for her, I realise that is all I have ever been - her wind up walking doll.
She doesn't ever notice me. Still. Never has.
Love me? No, she will never like me let alone love me.
But maybe I can get her to notice me. That I am real.
What can I do?
Smother her baby?
It has just come to me that when I did it to Kingsley, I was really doing it to her. He wasn't walking or talking. Or

# IN A PLACE OF DISCONNECTION

being clever. So it was easy.   Smothering her for not loving me.

So I am wondering whether I should do that to her baby. Doing bad things to her is what always got me noticed before, wasn't it? Why did I forget that?

Smother her baby?
Yes, that's it.
Put a pillow over her face.

# Pamela Pickton

GUY AND DOLL

Loretta looked with irritation at the costume dolls on the kitchen window sill. The girl doll was leaning on the boy again. Angrily, she propped the doll upright and began cleaning out the fridge.

It was the dependence of the doll she despised – leaning on the man like that. She rubbed fiercely at a stubborn mark. She loathed seeing any woman weak, dependent. And she hated herself for being so dependent on Michael. They`d had another row last night, she and Michael, a big row. Teeth clenched, she ruthlessly threw away half-used packets of this, not quite finished tubs of that. It had been the same old row, treading a well-worn track. How she wanted a baby, none came, and she blamed him.

He always said it was probably his fault; that illness he'd got while working in the Middle East before they met. She didn't believe it. She asked him to get a proper check-up, saying he was using the illness as an excuse for not going for tests. Secretly Loretta feared he didn't want a baby – perhaps he didn't even want her – and somehow, subconsciously, that was affecting things.

Having finished the fridge, she began to re-polish every inch of the already spotless kitchen.
Wiping the windowsill, she picked up first the boy doll, then the girl – the boy with the black trousers and frilly shirt, the girl with her braided skirt and crisp, embroidered apron. Her mother had brought them back from one of her holidays. She was always bringing back little kick-knacks, always going on foreign holidays. Loretta and Michael never went anywhere exciting. That was another cause of endless arguments. Michael always claimed he'd been put off far away places and heat - by that same old illness. Loretta said it was really because they couldn't afford it. And what was he doing with the money and whom was he spending it on?

# IN A PLACE OF DISCONNECTION

The next morning, Loretta stumbled bleary-eyed into the kitchen after a sleepless night. The first thing her eyes fell on was the pair of dolls. Were they looking at her? Last night had been  the worst row they`d ever had. She knew she had been cold towards Michael lately, saying she saw no point in making love since it didn't lead to a baby. This time Michael had actually accused her of not wanting a baby at all. She was just using all this because she was frigid. She always had been. What did she want him for anyway? She was just a little girl wanting a daddy to look after her.. A little girl whose mother was still bringing her dolls. She was probably secretly taking the pill.

Long after he eventually slept, Loretta had lain awake alone in the dark, staring into the blackness. Now, she looked at the dolls with a bitter sideways glance.  She seemed to hate  those dolls. Yet why should she? She'd always liked the other presents Mummy brought her. She'd always given Loretta pretty things.  It had just been the two of them for so long since Daddy died, and with no brothers or sisters.

Was it that the dolls were alone – no baby costume doll – or that they sometimes seemed so solidly, eternally together.  She didn't really know but today, as she looked, the boy doll looked so sure of himself.  And the girl doll? Well, weak really, a bit pathetic.  Irritated by their gaze, Loretta grasped the boy fiercely and moved him away from the girl, standing him on the spice rack on the opposite wall.

That night Michael didn't come home.

Again Loretta lay awake.  She didn't really think of the dolls at first but Michael had never done this before. Maybe it was work and he'd forgotten to tell her.  Maybe he was ill.  Maybe it was an accident.  Maybe she'd hear something  in the morning.  More likely, she thought next morning, he was sulking because of that foul row they'd had. Punishing her. She thought the girl doll looked wistful and the boy looked accusing. She told herself not to be ridiculous.

As the days went by, Michael didn't return or send a message. Loretta felt stranger. She felt so alone in the house with only the dolls looking at her. One morning she came into the kitchen to find the boy doll lying face down on the workshop. That day, out at the shops, she overheard some gossip. It was in a crowded supermarket and the women didn't see her but they were the wives of Michael's colleagues. She heard then saying Michael was ill. Loretta went home and looked hard at the dolls, wondering.

For several days she stayed in the house, wandering from room to room, lying awake at night. Wondering and thinking. Then one morning she stood the boy upright on the window sill again and pushed the girl doll into the drawer. Then she went up to the box of Christmas decorations in the spare bedroom and brought down the Christmas tree fairy. She had tinselly, blonde hair and was the same size as the costume doll. Loretta stood her beside the boy doll.

A few days later she heard a rumour that Michael had gone off with this secretary. Abroad!

For several days she looked at the dolls, wondering at her power. Confident, she stuffed the fairy doll back in her box and stood the girl doll next to the man on the window sill. They hadn't been together like that since Michael left. All day, she prepared food and cleaned the house. Then, in the evening, triumphant, she went upstairs to change, dress up, put on perfume.

She heard the car crunch over the gravel in the drive as she ran downstairs. She opened the kitchen door to pour herself and Michael a celebratory, homecoming drink.

# IN A PLACE OF DISCONNECTION

And as she heard his key turn in the door behind her, she saw the girl doll lying on the floor...

With her head snapped off!

# Pamela Pickton

THE WOODEN DOLL

Once, he was going to make rocking horses and try to sell them at places like Harrods. He was, well… a kind of lover I suppose, an artist, a teacher of art in Adult Education and in his view a failed painter. He had never sold much of his work, which was why he was looking for sidelines. At one time there was a fashion for whole walls, outside walls of buildings, to be painted like a vast external mural. Then, he longed to be commissioned to do one of those.

Next, he had the idea of making and marketing those little wooden artists' dolls, the ones that are all joints so that painters can move them about and draw the human figure in any position without the use of a human model.

Sometimes I felt he did not want a real live woman, maybe he wished that I was a wooden doll. On holiday I walked behind him, in Florence, while he enjoyed everything, but ignored me, not speaking.

'What are you thinking,' I said, standing behind him as he gazed at a painting.
'What are you doing? Feeling?'
'Love,' he said, 'Just love.'
Love, I thought, for this ancient face in ancient oil on ancient canvas. What about the real flesh and blood girl walking behind you? You never say you love her.

He was a lonely, unsociable man. His old friend, also an artist, who lived near him, told me, 'He doesn't want people, I can tell you...'
She must guess I'm always hoping he'll marry me, I thought, and is trying to warn me.
'...You know those tiny bushes – little trees – he has planted all along his front wall? Well he told me how tall they will grow,' she continued. One day they will totally block out his light. Block out the world from his view.'

# IN A PLACE OF DISCONNECTION

Her words came back to me when he talked of his photographic slides one day. He took a lot of photographs, doing his own developing, and using these to paint from.

'I may be alone,' he said, 'but I can get out my slides, and there, I have all those people.'

He retired early from the college – he said to paint, and we parted about this time. He had a flat in town, near me, as well as the country place near his painter friend. Now, he would keep only the cottage, which was in a village sixty miles away. He had never made the dolls or the rocking horses, but he told me now that he was going to make a life-size artists' doll and it would sit on his sofa.

Company without effort or commitment, I thought. I pictured him moving that doll, manipulating it, making it be just what he wanted it to be - as he had done with me. I had stayed with him in his cottage many times over the years and so could imagine the trees grown tall and his enclosed world with the doll looking at him, waiting for revenge.

'I have a strange feeling about his place, that village,' I told a friend and I went on to tell her of my belief in what I call loops of time. All the roads we do not take and all the lives we might have lived, maybe some part of us does travel in those ways, and so I wrote to him at the end of the relationship.

'Maybe another me will always be beside you, down there, in the country, with you.'

'And, I have another strange idea,' I tried to explain to the friend. 'It's a bit like the loops of time, but a bit different. It comes over me whenever I am some place where I go a lot. I first felt it at our nearest zoo, when I was forever taking my children there. I stood looking at the model village they had and thinking, it feels like I am always here.  So maybe I always am, and in all the places I visit frequently, his college, a swimming pool, your living room.

'So, do you see, I could be in that village in the country. In two ways, imprinted on the scene by habit, or because to live there is one path down which I might have gone.'

I heard he had died.  My friend told me.  She still went to the art collage where he had taught and they had heard the news.In fact he had been killed, clubbed to death.

It was the doll, I thought.  Behind that window, hidden by the tall trees, it got up one day from that sofa, walked over to where he sat in his armchair looking at his slides, or dozing – he often dozed in the day – and clubbed him to death: its revenge for keeping it trapped for so long.

I had always known it would.

Then the police came for me.

'I have not been to that village for ten years,' I said.

'But you were seen,' they said.  'People remembered you from when you did stay there. His neighbour, the other artist; she recognised the description of the woman seen and gave us your name.

'You were seen going past his window, his trees, trying to look in his window, every night.  All these years.'

# IN A PLACE OF DISCONNECTION

THE ADMIRERS

Look at her now, in the picture, in her garden framed by honey-suckled walls and spreading trees. Inside the frame, the spilling flowers and darting fish pond. And there she is in the middle, our lady, surrounded by her pets - ten cats, isn't it?

She is sitting on the grass with some flowers she has been picking, massed into a basket; little flowers and plants or perhaps they are herbs? The cats are all around her, on the grass, some on her lap and one on her shoulder. They lick her hand and rub against her and she pets them all.

Anyone would think she had no other admirers.

In fact, she has always had a stream of gentlemen callers, admittedly, never the same one for long. Mr. Black, somebody Colman, Alexander ... They come and they go, but what does it matter? They were all such fine fellows, all such elegant and suitable suitors. And why shouldn't she have so many admirers, she of the smooth and slinky beauty?

'Men,' she tells her friends, 'they always go.'

She looks up now, her little heart shaped face alert beneath her cap of shiny black hair, and her slant eyes move towards the house as she hears the doorbell. The cats jump away, meowing with complaint, as she pads indoors on the quiet little ballet pumps she always wears. Leisurely she walks in, as though she expects her caller to wait and she opens the door to a man. Kim, or is it Kurt?

'Come in, come in,' says Katrina, smiling and opening the door just enough for him to get through. She allows just a small embrace and then motions him to sit on the low cushioned chair, curling herself up on the floor in front of him. She folds her legs, in their clingy black satin, and the others come in from the garden and sit either side of her, facing him. She smiles across at the man, she likes him. She feeds him weak tea and then he says he will take her out to eat.  He orders steak, which is his favourite, and wine, but she will take only the fish course.

'Animals,' she yawns, licking her fingers, 'I love animals too much.'

'But fish,' he laughs, and she explains how that is different.  Fish are not cooped up like most  animals bred for man and, of all, are surely the most 'free range'.
'...It is more natural.'
She smiles a bewitching smile, stirring her ice cream to soft milk.  She likes his brown hair and curly beard, with little auburn highlights.

The next week, 'come in, come in,' she smiles a broader smile and opens the door wider. Wearing a cool grey siren suit, she enfolds him in her arms and the cats encircle them. He kisses her.
'Stroke my hair instead,' she says, and he strokes it.
'What shall we eat?'  He asks.  'Shall I go out for something?'  She chooses fish and chips and throws her chips for the birds.
'You shouldn't do that,' he says, 'you shouldn't encourage the birds. Your cats will get them.'
'Well, why not?' One cat nuzzles her feet and she picks it up, 'Why, it is only natural, after all...
'You would.'

Now, it is the next time and observe her waiting for him, getting ready for her admirer. The cats watch her from the silken eiderdown and the curly rug. Just one sits on her lap and another on the dressing table - sharing the mirror with her. She talks to them about her caller in a soft, contented murmur, while she files and files again her

# IN A PLACE OF DISCONNECTION

long, red nails. Then she laughs, pushing the cats off playfully and springs up to look in the full-length mirror, running her hands all over her silky outline. Today she is wearing a white playsuit, all in one, with a zip up to her only ornament; a little black necklace of a ribbon. The cats leap to attention from all directions and line up beside her, in silent adoration.

Then he arrives and tells her how beautiful she is and how much loved. He covers her with kisses and says he is gasping. Gasping for what? She brings him tea with ice-cold milk. 'It is so hot,' she says. He is tired on this hot day and wants to lie down. He wants to take her with him and lie down on her big, soft bed. She pushes all the cats out and they mew outside the door while he throws himself upon her greedily.

'Stroke my back first,' she rolls over. She wriggles and writhes, 'Oh, stroke me all over.'

After this, they are warm together, and he visits every day. They sit outside with low bowls of chilled herb soup and she cradles his head on her lap, stroking the beard that is reddening with the sun. He tells her of his life:
'I go home every week,' he warns her, 'and sometimes my work takes me away.'
Then he talks of broken dreams and many failures; of his sense of impending age.

'It's your unhealthy life,' she tells him, 'your diet, which is all-wrong. All that steak and wine and coffee. Poisoning your system and addling your brain. You should eat more good food and lead a more natural life. You'll be dead by the time you are fifty.'

She takes him climbing and for long walks, and after they lie together in the late summer sun.

# Pamela Pickton

'Yes,' she muses, as the sun beats down on his reddening sideburns and she tickles under his chin with grass.

'Yes, you would only be dead by the time you were fifty anyway…'


The next day he finds her curled up asleep in the garden, wearing a white dress splashed with brown and black and grey.

'Let me make tea,' he says, but he makes it too hot. She tips hers into the saucer to drink, feeling his eyes on her.

'You worry too much,' she laughs. 'I've told you. Be more relaxed.' One of the cats shares the tea with her from the saucer. 'Look at my lovelies. Not a care in the world.'

Later, she serves him soup. 'My own recipe,' she smiles, her eyes glinting, but he cannot manage the spoon in the low dish.

'It's good for you,' she laps hers and licks her lips, 'Full of cream.' She cups her hands round the bowl and tips it up. 'Drink it like this,' she says, 'from the bowl, that's how soup like this should be enjoyed.'

'Now you've made me get it all over me,' he says. But he gurgles quite happily as he licks and wipes around his gingering whiskers.

'Never mind,' she says stroking him. Never mind, Kurt. Or is it Kit…?


The autumn leaves are blowing and the cats rush round with the wind. There is the front door of her house, the wall and the tall hedge of bushes. The cats know she is coming. She has been out and it is as though they have been searching the world for her. And as her long, black legs come into view, they bound and leap from all corners. Some crowd on gate and wall, waiting, wailing and purring. A few stand stiffly by the door, like a sentry guard.

She strides along silently on her little black feet, and her arms clutch many parcels, many things. Against the wind,

# IN A PLACE OF DISCONNECTION

she has enclosed her hair inside a black furry cap, which buttons under her chin, and from it her little face smiles out as she sweeps through the gate, the cats milling and tumbling around her.

'Wait my darlings,' she says, unloading the shopping, 'be patient, Blackie, Sandy, Soot...' Then she serves them fish in low bowls and pours herself creamy milk.

'I have a new admirer now,' she tells them drinking hungrily:  Mr Tomson, Tom, or is it Tim?

'He's coming this evening; I have a lot to do'. She is padding round the kitchen as she speaks, putting things away. She looks into a mirror, preening, fluffing up her hat-squashed hair and licking it into place.

See her in the garden this evening now. Framed by wind blown trees and leaf-clothed floor. She lazes on the lawn, enjoying a snatch of evening sun and wearing a new, clingy robe of velvet brown. She smiles at the cats asleep around her.

Did he tire of her, or she of him?

'My new friend will be here soon,' she tells them.  'But none of you need fear. I will never love anyone as I love you, for only you are the faithful, the true admirers.'

'A new friend,' she tells them as the doorbell rings and she yawns and uncurls to answer it. They stand up and form a line watching her. Waiting. Adoring.

Look at them all around her.
Eleven cats, isn't it?

# Pamela Pickton

## STILL LIFE

Laura opened the gate with relief.  She was exhausted after the long climb up the hill from the station in this heat, and was glad to be back in her new home.  Well, not new of course, but new to her.  Pretty as a picture - roses round the door even - and looking as peaceful as a still life painting.  How dare those villagers mutter tales of it being haunted!  Probably some of them had wanted the old cottage for themselves. Well, they hadn`t managed to scare Laura off and now she smiled with pride as she turned the key in the front door, watching her country gingham curtains flutter behind the leaded windows.

All the gloomy forebodings had been hilarious when you thought about it. They had arrived only a few days ago by train, she and the children, as most of their things were following on later. They had rucksacks with basics including sleeping bags, and the cat in its basket, and most of the furniture would arrive the next day.  From the station, an ancient looking man had driven them to the cottage in a truck he boasted was the local taxi; and just before he drove off again he warned Laura that many had come to live here, but none had stayed, and that the locals avoided this end of the lane.

Laura remembered his words with a moment`s fear as she went into the kitchen to make herself a drink and heard a funny bumping  sound upstairs. She pulled herself together and laughed. It was the cat, of course. She put the kettle on the gas stove and began washing up the breakfast things that she had left in the rush to get the children to the train that would take them to their school. Weekly boarding had seemed the best solution after all that had happened, at least for the moment.

  Washing up, she looked out of the kitchen window to the wilderness of a garden. There at last lay the peace she had craved after the rat race of city life – and her divorce.

# IN A PLACE OF DISCONNECTION

Her life for a time frozen, suspended - another 'still life' she laughed - she had to look forward and build something new. And what better way to start than by reclaiming the garden, where already she could see her cat was at home. There it was, stalking a bird.

The cat? Laura gasped as again she heard the noise upstairs, and her heart began to race as she realised she had been watching the cat at play for some minutes. Oh, stupid. Just muffled noises. Those kids had left the radio on again. She poured her coffee. It was going to be lonely here. She had ended up with little money for a property, she needed seclusion and there was no school within walking distance. She must keep herself occupied while she got over things, try to get strong, then find a job and make some friends. For the moment, there was enough to fill her time, Laura thought, going out into the hallway to unpack more boxes.

Irritated by the gabbling sounds upstairs, yet too busy to go upstairs to switch off the radio, she suddenly became aware of another noise. Her cat was at the front door, mewling oddly, so she opened the door and bent to stroke him. It was then she felt the first prickle of real fear as her fingers sensed the raised fur before he spat and darted past her into the living room. Again Laura calmed herself. She was being silly. Everyone knew that cats were strange creatures and could react in all sorts of odd ways to house moves. It would take time for him to settle, that was all. She went back into the kitchen where her coffee had gone cold and turned the gas on again. But sitting down with her cup she had another fright. As she looked out of the window a tall tree was waving, it seemed threateningly towards her, in an inky sky. Strange when it had been so bright even when she let the cat in and the weather forecast had just said....

The radio!

# Pamela Pickton

As Laura stared at the radio beside her on the kitchen table, the gurgling noises upstairs grew louder.

She really must pull herself together, she thought. Fancy listening to an old man, and she would not be frightened off by the jealous villagers who everyone knew always hated outsiders. Of course! It was a television on, in the kids' bedroom. Now it was whistling because the programme had finished. She ought to go and turn it off. The devils! It was always the same; the radio forever left on, wearing out batteries. She had promised them their own television set to make up for all the upheavals.

Unpacking again, she resolved to get out of the house for part of the day. Loneliness was making her edgy. The kitchen tap was dripping and it was jarring at her brain. She tried to ignore it. Was that a chuckle upstairs? Well, either another programme had started, or she was imagining things. Laura worked quickly, fiercely, but both noises were getting at her now.
Drip, drip, drip.
Mumble, mumble, mumble.
She must unwrap one more cup, one more cup, one more cup…
Smash.

Her best rose china, her own fault for getting so tense. She marched to turn off that blooming tap.

The radio was near the taps now, on the draining board. Now, who the devil? Crazy! Again she had to tell herself off. All the stress had made her a bit forgetful lately. She had just forgotten moving it, that was all. What could she do? Ring for something to be delivered? Just hearing another human voice would keep her sane. Who? What? Laura moved heavily into the front room, hoping the cat would tolerate a cuddle now. They both needed comfort. But where was he? She did not remember seeing him come out. A pulse began throbbing at her temple. Then

# IN A PLACE OF DISCONNECTION

there was a bang at the front door. Laura froze. She had been told there was no postal service so far out, and when she forced herself to look on the mat there was nothing, nor any retreating shadow through the side window.

Perhaps her friends? They knew her address. Special delivery, a parcel left outside? Flowers?

She opened the door. On the step, a dead bird.

Laura's hand flew to her throat; then, angrily, she kicked the bird out of sight. But as she went back into the living room she tried to rationalise why that had been such a shock. The divorce, the move, they had made her sensitive. Some wretched cat had put the bird there. As if anyone else would...

But as she looked out of the front window she was almost paralysed by the sight of the blazing sun and motionless bushes. Why, only a moment ago when she had been turning off the tap...

She ran back to the kitchen where a black sky seemed to mock her. Still she tried to be rational. It was that time of year: heat and storms, patchy changeable weather, rain in places. But her breath was coming faster now. Was that a moaning she could hear upstairs now? No, only the background hum all televisions make occasionally. But as she crouched amidst the clutter in the hall, she had to admit that she was putting off going upstairs to see to it. And as her gaze wandered wearily to a family photograph sticking out of one of the packing cases, the voices rose to a scream in her ears.

Her own face had been scribbled out.

Those wicked children. Trying out their new pens before they left. On anything. Without looking.

# Pamela Pickton

She was nearly shouting aloud now. Then new hope came with the approaching throb of a car engine. If only someone would come. To see a face. Talk to somebody. It must be going to stop here, surely? A visitor. Or a delivery van. That was it. They had promised to come and...

And her last pretence trailed away with the wheels of civilisation that had already rumbled past and faded into the distance.

For there was no phone.
Nor even any electricity.

And the television set had not yet been delivered.

# IN A PLACE OF DISCONNECTION

TO REACH THE SKY

There was a place where water flowed, with moss and seaweed like plants, and rocks that glowed with a fluorescent light.  But of course there was never any sun.  Almost everywhere was dark, gloomy, functional, places of work; communal residences, a few attempts at sport and leisure centres.

Well, it was new, a new city, a new country, built with difficulty, under pressure and almost without plan.  To the stream and to the blessed waterfall, people came in allocated turns for half an hour's respite.  It would almost have been a holiday if only they could have fabricated a sun.

But how do you have a sun without a sky?

It had all happened suddenly, was it true that they had ignored the forebodings?  For fifty, perhaps a hundred, years the words 'population explosion' had rumbled like distant, safe, thunder around the outskirts of reality. Few saw any threat as the words took concrete meaning; more blocks of flats, enforced sharing, eviction of single occupiers of whole houses, and finally the disappearance of all open land.

Surely it would be all right in the end?

After five years of ignored, unbelievable, warnings, the political bomb fell like the declaration of war.  All, but the oldest and necessary experts, were driven to a new life.

Underground.

Many had died of the shock, most had forgotten.  Life was better here, after all, than in the crowded world above.  Besides, the exodus had been thirty years ago now.  A great number of the dwellers of darkness had been born here; they had never seen the sky. And, naturally, with each passing year, death brought vacancies above, especially for anyone offering great skill. Therefore, spirits were high. The older people, still stunned with disbelief, dreamed of another answer, a better plan. The young bent all their energies on striving for higher qualifications.

For the young, there was one other way of reaching the sky. The world above was wearying of the aged, and those in charge recognised the morale boosting necessity of young faces in the community. So any young person could put their name on the lost list to ascend. Provided they were irrevocably sterilised.

Such was the dilemma which now faced June and Gary as they sat beside the stream, enjoying what was neither a spring, summer, nor winter holiday. There were no seasons in this realm of caves and burrows, only heating, air conditioning and artificial light. Indeed, this was the cause of Gary's discontent. He was older than June and could remember, albeit faintly, picking daisies for his mother, trudging through snow, and flying his kite, high high in the sky.

June was only eighteen and knew no more than stories, of splashing waves, tall rustling trees and fluffy white clouds. She could scarcely imagine it. But she knew what Gary wanted and she loved him desperately. She longed to have a child of her own, their child, but she could not bear to see him so restless. And she knew that if it came to it, where he went, she would follow.

Still, she wept now, by the water, thinking of her unborn babies, putting off the decision, not giving him the final answer. And he comforted her with kisses, with incredible legends of the earth's multitudinous, various creatures, and mountains whose tops went beyond sight into the clouds. Urgently, he pressed his belief that the

# IN A PLACE OF DISCONNECTION

nightmare would end. There could be planetary evacuation. The operation might after all be reversed.

They clung together desperately, as time ran out and he must return to medical lectures, she to her nursing course. They rarely met alone anymore. Not since he had become so obsessed with reaching the sky, for there was always the chance of that final damnation.

And who could leave a baby behind?

But when their turn for the stream was in the late evening period, and many who could come were too tired, then Gary and June found themselves almost alone, between the rocks, in the shadows. Too much alone. Then, she would turn in his arms wearily, and his gentle embrace became fierce.

The memory was sweet now, as she left him and hurried from the place of water. She smiled and remembered those secret times, for then all heartbreak was forgotten. But she mustn't daydream like this. She must face facts. Sit down seriously and think. Soon he would qualify. His name was high on the list. They could miss their turn if they were not married, and organised. Tomorrow she would make up her mind, or at least in the next few days. But she needed him to help her and suddenly he was never there. In the weeks that followed he was always busy, fighting for improvements underground, making his voice known and of course daily inspecting the new vacancies. June heard vaguely of big meetings, but took little interest. All she knew was that she scarcely saw him. Panicking, she pictured a new girl, one who was willing. Then, one day he came to her, briefly, smiling and reassuring. It wouldn't be long now. Everything was going to be all right after all. But his air of mystery frightened her, and his visit left her sick with worry.

Sick. Yes, sick.

# Pamela Pickton

Slowly the truth dawned. Faint, as though in a dream, she hunted for him but could not find him. Must she bear it all alone? Then one day she caught sight of him but in the distance, in a crowd, marching. He could only wave and shout as he was carried from her by the jostling, excited mob.

'Only a month. Wait. Wait.'

Only a month?

She must move fast to do what she must do. At least now it would be two ordeals over in one.

And afterwards, alone having told no one, she lay weak and despairing, when suddenly he burst into her room. Jubilant. Reviving. He looked so happy and she held his hand to her wet face, as she cried her sad story.

It was then he froze, slumped down by her bed, his head in his hands. He stepped quickly to the door and spoke with his back turned, before walking away. June listened to the determined voice, knowing she would not keep him even if she could. He had aimed for the sky, while she had thought she was simply killing two birds with one stone. Now she knew she had killed all birds, and would never see one fly. Nor would there ever be that oasis of love, not even in the place where water flowed.

For there had been far reaching sickness in the place where fresh winds blew. Numbers were halved and sad old hearts were failing.

Most qualified hopefuls, next in line to ascend, were now struck off the list, for they had early prepared themselves in the manner dictated. Gary, who had waited for her yes, now left her broken while he was whole. He was first on the list.

# IN A PLACE OF DISCONNECTION

The old world wanted more than technicians now.

It wanted the young, the strong, and the healthy

And those able to give child.

# Pamela Pickton

THE DRAGON

They called her the old Dragon, the matron of the home. And no wonder, Nell thought, throwing the pots into the sink, breaking a few on purpose. Always bullying and bossing, making everyone's life a misery; a tyrant, a dragon, one who was feared and placated lest she consumed them with fire. A dragon's breath of flames could not be more dreaded than matron's wrath, directed at the old people, the staff, and most of all at Nell.

Nell, the kitchen hand, the dogsbody, the nobody. Orphaned, deserted, let down so many times. It seemed that fate had kicked her into the mud, and then ground in its heel. She didn't think she had the energy to struggle up again. And why bother? She would only be knocked down again. The old dragon knew this and played on it. Nell never complained to anyone. And if she did where else could she go? Her youth and chances of marriage were nearly over. The matron had an easy slave. That was why Nell was washing up now. She never got a Sunday off. The old ladies were sleeping. The doctor was on call. The dragon was out and the staff were cut to a bare minimum. Barely legal, it sometimes seemed to Nell, especially when one was called home on an emergency and the dragon had no contingency plans. And anyway, while Nell skivvied all Sunday afternoons, she knew the few on duty took this time when the residents slept to plug into their music, paint their nails or do some texting. No, she never got a day off but it wasn't worth complaining. There was nowhere Nell wanted to go anyway.

When she had first earned her living, had time and money to spare, she had tried dances and parties like other girls but had found it a nightmare. She was tongue tied, awkward and clumsy and totally incapable of dancing. She knew that it was all tension. The dragon had taught her that. Many times she had been bursting with a head full of anger, yet could not utter a sound. At those times she felt like a bomb that needed the pin taking out.

At dances, it had been the same tight feeling. Like a toy, a spinning top, whose string had come tangled and knotted so that it would not undo. Yet, alone, in the secrecy of her room, Nell danced. Her string unwound, she was released. She loved the abandonment of dancing. But she longed to share it, and she longed to be seen as her real self.

Finishing the washing up, she wiped her hands on her apron and removed the regulation cap from her scraped back, high-knotted hair. She could never release all her trapped passions while living here. Daily, the dragon hammered her further into the floor. But, if she were to escape, would she ever recover?

She almost believed, now, that she was the fool, the careless idiot. She was the prisoner of the home, the old dragon, and herself. But at least for a few hours, she was alone. She switched on the kitchen radio and threw her apron across the room as her ears caught the sound of 'The Stripper'. How she loved that tune. Slowly at first she began to move, looking over her shoulder, hesitating. Then shyly, letting her hips sway, she wriggled out of her cardigan. Still bolder, she let her shoulders join in, lifted her chest and held up her chin. The music rose to a crescendo as she flung her arms wide. And it ended as she leapt across the room, leaning breathless against the sink, wishing it could go on.

Now there was only talking. She switched the radio off. Yet, surely, there was the clash of cymbals again, or was she going mad? No, it was outside, a band, and coming this way. Oh, how she loved a band. Before she knew what she was doing, she had left her post and was watching the band approach. Guiltily, she felt her feet tapping as if they did not belong to her. And, as the band passed, it somehow pulled her, as though she had no will. At a distance first, she followed haltingly, but soon found she had edged up. It was then she knew that she must stay with the marchers. It had been a joke. She had meant to go back, but now all that mattered in the world was to try and match their rhythm. Desperately, Nell tried to keep in step and still stumbling, found the band had led her out of the street, out of the town itself.

First, they came to a country village and a May Fair, where the band never stopped marching, though it twirled with the others round the ribboned pole.
Then, out of the village and away. Up hill and down hill, never tiring. She was stronger now. Yes, and in time. At last, in time. Occasionally, she missed a beat. But she was getting it. Her feet were surer. And somehow she had worked her way to the middle. Well, why not? Nell strode on unbelieving. She was holding a drum. Perhaps someone had passed it to her, for she was part of them now, one with them and they drew her ever onwards. It was too late to go back. The band would not let her, and why should she?

Nell at the sink no longer existed. Had she forgotten that her real name was Eleanor? She unknotted her trapped hair and let it fly out behind her, while the throbbing drums and the clashing cymbals hypnotised her, and the swaying movements of those in front drew her magically on into the night. For hours, they seemed to be marching through a jungle and the distant answering tom-tom did not surprise her. Sometimes, between dark shiny leaves, a spear could be seen or a watching face, striped in paint. Faster, faster they marched and she was aware of danger, aware of fear, but they did not look back.

Then, they were out of the jungle at last and day had dawned. With relief, they found themselves now mixed up in a carnival. Clowns with large cardboard heads jostled her. The sounds were clashing, laughing, thrilling.

# IN A PLACE OF DISCONNECTION

Why, she was walking taller now. Streamers caught round her hair, and she danced and twirled. A lady in medieval costume brushed her arm, a lady tripped by wearing a conical hat with a scarf floating from it. It was then she decided – no, I am Eleanora.

But the band wove itself out of the carnival. Still it seemed they must march. The music beat louder, she pounded her drum. Yet her feet seemed lighter than ever. And, yes, somehow she seemed to have worked forward almost to the front. Now, pagodas were in sight and there was a tinny music and strange people lining the streets. There seemed to be cheers, even adoration and it seemed to be for her. She looked down at herself.

Now she could forget the past, the home, the matron, even Nell. Of the future she had no knowledge but it held no fear.

She could be in control. She would be King of any domain just because she believed in herself. She could control any situation, control her own life.

Because today she led the parade. Proudly.

In the figure of a dragon.

# Pamela Pickton

DREAMS COME TRUE

Driving to work below grey skies, George Watson's face showed none of its usual Monday morning strain. His thin lips were parted in expectancy, and his thinning pate held proudly in hope. Stupid hope, he half knew, yet he just had to see. To see what the day brought forth, to see if the Fortune Teller's words came true. Crazy, to hang on to something – no more than a joke he supposed.
' Madam Zola ', probably a postmistress dressed up for fun, a frustrated actress or even a man, next job Father Christmas.

Fortune Tellers! Always there, always at fairs and on piers, crouched in their tents. Shadowy, black draped, like spiders to which endless victims never ceased to be drawn like flies. And he  - who had nobody to take to a fair or to the seaside, no family and for the last five years, not even a girl friend. Not since Jenny.

Then, in the pub on Saturday there was the mystery woman hired by the village for the carnival, and the bets and the daring and the men egging him on. The Fortune Teller in the corner, in the shadows. Dark shadows but for the glinting baubles and beads. Nothing real but her eyes, as he got nearer. Her hand spread in rings and bangles like a veil up to her eyes and above them, ending in earrings that might hypnotise, a brilliant silk scarf. Gold and green and white and black, and were there little red bits? Or was that her hair? Those eyes, which fixed his dithering footsteps, drew him to her, glittering and looking at him as though she had known him all her life.

Her pronouncement like a benediction, a blessing, reaching to the very core of his hopeless middle age: 'On Monday.'

` On Monday you will make love.`

# IN A PLACE OF DISCONNECTION

Was it foolish to believe?  Her last words to him had been, 'you must have faith.' Surely her magic had reached this far, for here he was, through the gates not once having sworn at the traffic.  Rather he had been watching every skirt that passed and wondering, who?

At his desk, he watched the grey skies unchanging and the clock ticking round to ten, to eleven, to nearly twelve. Was he supposed to make an effort, or was it all going to happen? He fidgeted in his chair, almost expecting one of the typists to rush in at any moment and claim him.

At twelve-thirty, since no damsel had dropped from the heavens, he cleared his throat and asked his secretary to come to lunch.  They hardly ever conversed and besides, she was older, rather prim, but who knew what heart beat beneath that knitted bosom? She had important shopping to do.  Well, he would go to his usual pub and maybe there... But after an hour of  trying to pluck up the courage to join the long legged smart girls perched on stools, he trod wearily back to the office, shaking.  A casual pick up - that had never been his style.

So he let himself remember Jenny, red haired Jenny who had been his secretary five years ago 'til she told him she could no longer have a job, or a man, because she was needed at home. With pain he remembered how quickly she had gone.  Had she ever given back his key?  He was beginning to give up when the tea lady's trolley rattled to his room and he thought, she's fat but she's jolly and she's beautiful in her way.

She was going to her bingo, and she couldn't come to the pictures.

The rain started as he left for home.  But he wasn't beaten.  There had been magic in the day.  Miss Arnold had blushed when he asked her to lunch.  He would ask her again, anyway.  The tea lady looked pleased and younger as she went rattling and singing down the corridor. He had seen people differently and prayed that his eyes would stay open. And there were six hours left, not to mention the young school teacher who shared his bathroom.

He passed the headscarf girl again. She lived hear him. Neighbours said she nursed an ailing mother. A shadowy figure, he always thought, rather drab. But today, because it was raining and because of the song in his heart, he offered her a lift. She sat in the back and hardly spoke, just blended into the shadows. Yet he found himself telling her of the Fortune Teller, laughing at his own expense.

At home, the school teacher was going to her yoga session but she smiled brightly and said she would love to come to dinner another time. Another surprise, he thought. She had always seemed too brash, so wrapped up in her busy life. And, quite happily, he let another hour slip away, opening a tinned pie. There was still time. He could go out. Monday was his launderette night. Even there, one could meet ones' destiny. But somehow, he could not move from the chair. He was warm and happy, wrapped in the memories of his different day and woken from a five-year death, to find new hopes of love.

'Tonight you will make love...' Oh Jenny, Jenny.
At half past eleven he switched out the light, not sad, not sad at all. He knew the old dame's spell would last forever. The joy of hope. And there was still half an hour, wasn't there?

When he woke, next morning, he knew what the words had meant. Her gift had been a dream. In his sleep a girl had slipped into his bed. In the dream it was dark, shadows hid her face and her hair was in the pillows. Yet their kisses were so sweet and their lovemaking seemed to contain all time, past and present and future. After all,

# IN A PLACE OF DISCONNECTION

the Fortune Teller had not said you will really truly make love, merely that he would.  And surely a dream, a dream like that, was good enough?

For it had seemed real enough, at the time.

George hugged the memory to him with the pillow.  And his fingers felt something hidden, something silky.

And the years ahead were no longer lonely but full of love.

As he kissed and kissed again the little scarf...
In which lay one red hair.

# Pamela Pickton

I DIDN'T KNOW YOU CARED

It was like so many marriages, Joyce supposed, a cartoon marriage with Harry asleep in front of the television each evening. A music hall joke of a marriage, in which Joyce spent her breakfast talking to silent newspapers. Like so many wives, she took to whimpering first, then to nagging.

Why couldn't they have a baby? Well, when were they going to start a family then? Could she have a dog in the meantime? A cat even? A budgie? Joyce was lonely and bored. When she tried a little part-time job, she became too upset by the other women's talk – of their new cars, their fitted kitchens, their holidays, and their children. So she went back to being a housewife again. She didn't really mind because the job had been boring anyway. She would have been quite happy in her life if only Harry had been different, given her just a little more attention or consideration.

They never went on holiday or even out for the day. They did not own a car. Harry said very little whenever she complained. He would not decorate the flat and took little interest when she did it herself. She knew he earned very little in the pharmaceutical factory where he worked. He had no go and was unlikely to get on, but she supposed she had always known that. No, it was his lack of interest that hurt, more than anything else. When she asked for a new dress, he would ask what was the matter with her old one? Then, if she appeared in something new, he seemed at a loss for anything to say.

The hopes of each fresh day were early ruined by the grunts and 'very nice dear's' from the eternal, unseeing newspaper. She began reading the newspaper herself, picking it up after he had gone to work. It was something to do, something else to think about. And the habit took her on to reading magazines. These intrigued her at first, with their claims of improving women's lives. 'Try a new hairdo, brighten your make-up, find a new hobby,' all the articles told her, 'if you want to make your man sit up.'

But oh, hadn't she tried everything, all the tricks in the book? What else could she do to win some attention, if not love, from her beloved Harry? For she did love him, though she did not bother to tell him so anymore. It would not matter to him. They lived in the same house but were strangers. All she wanted was some warmth to come across that breakfast table, but there was no close communication at all. Joyce felt left out in the cold, and wondered why Harry had married her. Never could she ask him that question, but how could she make him take notice?

Her magazines gave her an answer - the magazine stories with their loves and heartbreaks and nearly always a solution. The happy endings annoyed her sometimes but the stories themselves gave her an idea, a plan to wheedle her own happy ending. She began to write magazine stories herself. She sent them in, and gradually, some were accepted. Joyce told Harry. He seemed vaguely pleased that she should have found herself a little hobby. Each time she had a story published she left the magazine lying around the flat, opened at the appropriate page. She did not know if Harry read them. She just hoped

The stories were about women who ran away or had affairs – anything to win the attention of their husbands. One husband, coming home earlier than usual from work, found his wife dancing alone to soft music, wearing her evening dress at four in the afternoon, because he never gave her occasion to wear it. One heroine secretly sent herself van delivered flowers, 'til the florist found out and began sending them himself. It was not until the stories touched on breakdown and suicide that Harry commented at all. From behind the newspaper, he remarked that her writing was making her morbid, shut up as she was all day. Why didn't she try jogging instead?

But she could not stop now. Her imagination carried her along on a tide of fantasies, of dreams. She could not give up hoping now. When she wrote of a neglected wife murdering her husband, friends laughed.

'You're such a meek soul,' they said, 'what in imagination you must have.'

'Harry's more likely to do himself in,' joked one, 'the way you've been getting at him in your stories. All those dangerous chemicals he works with.'

The story in question was obviously one that Harry had read. One supper time, soon after it was published, Joyce looked at her husband as she put a forkful of casserole into her mouth and he actually smiled at her across the table.

'I switched our plates,' he laughed, 'just in case.'

He was so nonchalant, she could scream.

Why wasn't he getting the message?

All the evening, while Harry snored in his armchair, Joyce sat seething. Why, if she really were to leave him, he would not care. It was then that she realised that perhaps she no longer cared either. Her writing had changed her. It filled her days and not only that, it had taken her out and about. She had met more people.Might she not meet another man? Besides, she now had some money of her own. She could make a new life.

During the next weeks, Joyce thought and planned. Yes, she would leave Harry. She would go far away. In fact, the other side of the world would not be far enough. She bought her ticket and packed in secret. Harry was not going to hurt her anymore.

On the day itself, she sat down with a cup of tea, to await her taxi to the airport. She switched on the radio, just to pass the time and caught the morning story. She usually

# IN A PLACE OF DISCONNECTION

listened to it but this morning she was too preoccupied. These last minutes were dragging and her mind was in turmoil as she sat with cup in one hand, bag in the other and suitcase at her feet. All ready to make flight.
But it was impossible to ignore the story.

The voice drifted into her consciousness. It was a story about a man whose wife was too demanding. He was a man with no confidence. He was too scared of failure to take driving lessons. Let alone take on the lives of children. He was shy, undemonstrative and awkward. In the end, it was only when his wife threatened to leave him that he declared himself. He had always loved her.

Joyce's cup smashed to the floor as the author's name was read out ..

.. and she remembered what she had put in his mid-morning flask.

# Pamela Pickton

## THE CENTRE OF ATTENTION

I always had a proper wedding, the full works – every time. Three times.  The fanfare, the triumphal march. And all dressed up.

Someone even said to me once, after my second marriage failed very quickly,
'Why did you marry him?  Fancy a wedding? Want to be a bride? `
The answer I did not like to give was, really, yes.

I know what it is all about, where it all came from, in my past. When I was a child, at infant school, every year at Christmas they played this game. A chair was set in the middle of the hall and it was meant to represent a Christmas tree. Then all the children were divided into three groups; some to be parcels, some to be candles and some to be Christmas tree balls. The candles had to hold their hands above their heads, stretched tight with the fingers tapering together to look like a flame. The balls had to bounce up and down, and the parcels had to cross their hands over their chests like string. Then, one by one the groups danced up to the chair and stood round it `til they stood around the 'tree' like decorations. The 'balls' bounced towards the tree too and then stood around it; the 'parcels' jumped staunchly, squarely to take their place, and the candles ran with their arms tapering like flames alight. In place and waiting for the final decoration.

Every year I was in the school, three years I think, we played the game every week for at least a month leading up to Christmas, and every time, a different girl was chosen to be the fairy doll. She came in at the last minute, when all the other decorations were in place and stood on the chair. The fairy doll on top of the tree.
I was always the parcel. Not once was I the fairy doll.

# IN A PLACE OF DISCONNECTION

And well, I don't think I have ever got over that hurt. That feeling of being passed over, of not mattering, of being put last. I was never made much of at home either. My parents seemed to be too busy for me, and it sometimes seemed that they had never wanted children at all. The best way I could describe it is to say I felt completely ignored. Not noticed, not first, and certainly not made to feel pretty and special.

And so I married three times and every time dressed in the full regalia  - a proper bride. Oh, I could not have the big balloon dress, the big meringue they call it now, and a veil every time. You can't when you are in your forties or more, can you?  And in the case of those early weddings, the second and third, well the reason for the re-marriage was divorce, so you are not necessarily going to get a 'church do', are you? And of course, you would be getting a divorce wouldn't you, if the main reason you married was to be a bride for the day? A queen for a day. No, the second time I wore the long  white number– fairly balloony – with only flowers in my hair. The next time I wore a short dress. But it was lacy - and still dreamy, in what they called a creamy ivory.

So I was the last to arrive when all the other decorations were in place - all the guests, in other words, in their seats, waiting, hushed and excited as they always are, aren't they?  The women anyway - to see what I would be wearing. Waiting for my grand arrival, grand entrance. The fairy doll on top of the tree. The centre of attention.

But there comes a time, doesn't there? Can you wear the white in your sixties, seventies or eighties?  If you remarry at those ages you wear the sensible smart day dress or the tweed suit, don't you? So I had to find a different way. Yes, I wore the day dress, the suit, and the discreet and sombre clothes. For my weddings... (I have had three twilight marriages to date). But there are other occasions.

# Pamela Pickton

It was easy really, easy as pie, plain sailing or however you want to put it. The first of the older bridegrooms I got to carry me over the threshold. Well, I didn't know he had a dicky heart, I swear it. The second, well I knew he had been warned off cream and stuff, cholesterol and all that, but I was only being kind giving him little bits of what he was always begging me for. I did protest, I do assure you, of course I did. Oh, I admit that I did sometimes forget, got a bit carried away when we had guests to dinner. I love cooking  and well, I was using my favourite recipes and old habits die hard, like adding the bit of extra cream to the goulash.

This last one, well I was lucky that's all, he was well known to be a bit doddery. Ten years older than me and well… on honeymoon he got a bit too near the edge of a cliff, I got carried away with love and passion and all that, and gave him too strong a hug I suppose.

So, first Archie, then Charles gave me my chance to show off again. And now Fred – his unknowing legacy - a contribution to my new fairy doll act.

Here I am, where I have been twice already before.

I always arrange the ceremonies for two o`clock, so I can go for the facial and the hairdo first.

For I am on view today, on days like this. I am all dressed-up – not white, or cream but pale beige or a soft gold. (Oh, yes, they were my darlings` favourite colours, though nobody else seemed to know it.)

All eyes on me, all dressed up, the last to arrive.
I walk in, the centre of attention.

Behind the coffin.

# IN A PLACE OF DISCONNECTION

## A CUP OF SUGAR

And to think it all began with a cup of sugar too.
I must tell my story, must write it down.
Whether I'll ever be able to get this to anybody I don't know.  But it feels a bit of a letter-in-a-bottle-to-be-thrown-out-to-sea, just to set it all down.
If she saw me going out with something bulky to post – well, I think she'd prise it from me. She is very good at taking something off you.
Yes, it began with a cup of sugar.  Something as simple and as neighbourly as asking to borrow a cup of sugar.

It was a bit soon, just two days after we'd moved in next door to her but she was so jolly, so blustery, that it just felt like the beginning of a mutually beneficial relationship.
I had thought that maybe she'd come to introduce herself, seeing her that first time on my doorstep; come to help, or invite us round for a meal while we were up to our eyes with the unpacking.

Then  out popped the empty cup from behind her back.
I was to remember that 'behind-the-back' bit.
'That's what neighbours are for,' she laughed as she went off with the cup now full of sugar.  Nice to have somebody other than your usual neighbour who barely says good morning surely, and we could both help each other out of a hole from time to time.

The sugar was back after a few days, but with it a request to borrow half a dozen eggs.  I didn't think about it much at the time.  She said she would give the eggs back on Friday; two days time when it was her shopping and housekeeping day.

They were not back on Friday and in the end I went next door to ask for them on Monday when I was running a bit short myself. She could only give me four 'til Friday and could she borrow some flour?  In view of what had

# Pamela Pickton

happened over the eggs I now stipulated that I wanted eggs and flour by the next weekend. The situation was still not really bothering me though. She had so many hungry mouths what with five children, husband and a mother, who seemed to live there half the time, that I guessed she just must have miscalculated what she needed.

Just disorganised I thought, and we settled into a pattern for the next six months where she borrowed small amounts of groceries or cleaning materials two or three times a week, usually brought them back later than promised and always with a request for the next item.

I think the first big mistake I made was soon after I moved in and she told me that the Head of the Milk Marketing Board was coming to see her because she had left unpaid so many milk bills. It was not my problem, I realise that now, but that was not how my psychology worked. If somebody tells me a problem, I always have to do something about it. So I lent her the money because I was envisaging her in prison. Not that unreasonable, I defend myself. What would have happened to the five children? Of course, she then had to pay me back and let some other bill go to do it. That was her life, I was beginning to realise, always robbing Peter to pay Paul. I couldn't see how you benefited, living like that. You would only be 'quids in' during the first week when you got something for nothing. Ever after that, anything you saved by not paying for it, had to be used for last week's debts. Perhaps she just enjoyed living on a knife's edge.

I was providing this woman's life style. When it was not the borrowing it was the baby minding. My two children were a bit older than any of hers and, with so many, the age range of hers went down to near babies. We could not afford to go out a great deal and when we did I paid a sitter. With her though the child minding was mostly daytime, as in her taking one of the children to a medical appointment and leaving the others with me.

'Just picked up a few things on my way,' she lied, seeing my face, when she was gone much longer than promised and clearly holding a full shopping bag behind her back. Then the excuses came about the delays, the buses and the rest. She had not only kept her appointment but had a good old shop on me too.

The bluff and bluster panic became a bit of a pattern to distract from what she was really doing. For example, once she knocked on my door and when I opened it she was looking over her shoulder. She was going to her dressmaking class and could she borrow my cotton, and the request was overshadowed by the constant jerking of the head and looking down the road for the imminent arrival of the car which was giving her a lift.

Do you see? The focus was so much on her not missing the car coming for her, that what she was actually doing – taking, using up, my cotton, because she was hardly going to bring a few yards back – was masked. That did upset me. If she had paid to join an evening class in dressmaking, why didn't she buy her own cotton? Getting a lift too. How many backs was she riding on?

Upset and uncared for, that was how I was beginning to feel, as the now regular routine seemed to be me knocking on her door for something she had promised me three days ago. And she would say she had forgotten about it! Suppose I had forgotten? She would have 'stolen' whatever it was. And I was beginning to realise that all the bluster, promises and comments about how good I was, when she came over with a request, meant absolutely nothing. Once she had got the thing and gone back home, I was not in her head anymore.

# Pamela Pickton

I guess my game must have been trying to get someone to like me but it was something else too. I learned early that she is religious, a practising, Catholic, and since I am not anything in particular I wanted to show her that I was a good holy person too. We sometimes visited each other for coffee and on one of those occasions she confided in me that she felt she had no real friends. Well, of course that shook me, as I considered myself a very good friend to her.

'Oh, Oh,' the bluster again as she realised what she had said and rallied, telling me that of course she counted me as one of her best friends.Didn't want to kill the golden goose, I realise now.

I was getting used to the bluster and ruses, and the acting. One Sunday she came into my kitchen looking awful and, after the usual pleasantries, confessed that she was depressed. I played the game and got it out of her: she was out of cigarettes (she smoked sixty a day). There was no cash in the house and hubby would not let her write a cheque or put any more on their Visa.
'In the doldrums,' was how she described herself.
'Why don't I lend you the money?' I suggested, and she said what a good idea, as if that had not been the object of the visit all along.

Just now and again I broke, snapped. One day she was on the doorstep again, telling me that 'Auntie' (her period) had come to visit rather early and could she borrow a 'bunny'.

'Oh I do hate it when people say borrow when they mean keep,' I burst out.
When I told my husband he said, 'well she's not exactly going to give it back, is she?'

You may wonder about my husband in all this. Well, mostly he did not know what was going on but also we

# IN A PLACE OF DISCONNECTION

had our own problems too. We were breaking up around this time.

Maybe that is why I took so much abuse. I did not have the emotional energy to say,` no`.It was around this time that she borrowed one of our suitcases for a weekend away. The handle came off and she said she would get in mended. Week after week I went in and week after week she was going to do it next week. She had this expense and then that expense. In the end my husband went in and came back defeated, talking of the bluff and bluster that had greeted him just as I always did. All her explanations and promises were in this very posh voice, I forgot to say, which made it all the more convincing.

Soon after that my husband left us and I forgot all about the suitcase. As he packed his bags he said he could have done with that case! ( Actually, I think it was my being so pathetic with the neighbour which had finally cracked our marriage). I remember the day after he went, she caught me as I was going out and asked for a fiver. I almost emptied my purse at her feet because there seemed no point in anything. What I did do was give her my last fiver and say I must have it by Tuesday. She promised, but of course come Tuesday she had forgotten all about it and did not have five pounds.

Now weakened and in an even harder up state I thought she might help me. For example, I was finding it difficult to manage the large garden that had been a wilderness when we moved in and, what with all our other problems, we had never got on top of it. This neighbour was a keen gardener and so was her mother when she was there. Mother, who being of retirement age worked away as a kind of relief housekeeper for half of every month, lived with them the rest of the time since, as the borrower put it, she had helped them to buy the house. Anyway, I asked if there were any cuttings she was throwing away and if so, could she throw them in my direction.

# Pamela Pickton

Meanwhile a pattern set  in which was more intense than anything up to now, as the borrowing became relentless. Each week she would come in with a list of normal household commodities, wanting half a pound of this, half a pound of that, two ounces of something else and a cup or two of liquids like vinegar, tomato sauce or washing up liquid. The following week those bits would be dutifully returned together with a list of all the things she had not borrowed last time and would need this week.  Almost every household item needed replenishing at least every fortnight and she could not manage that. So she bought what she could and borrowed the rest, returning last week`s pinch of spice say, while borrowing this week`s cup of baking powder..  So it might be flour, custard powder, soap powder one week and then gravy powder, bleach, icing sugar, salt, the next.

They weren't always such long lists and it might be only a drop of vanilla essence and two spoonfuls of curry powder.  Perhaps because I was preoccupied with my own worries in my newly divorced state, I did not keep a proper check on it all.  I never paid much attention or kept copies of the lists, but I was aware in some part of my consciousness that not everything came back every time.

I missed reading my women's magazines that I could not longer afford, and knew that she bought two every week, so I asked if she could pass hers on to me.  After all, finished-with magazines and garden cuttings don't cost anything. I still believed she was my friend, you see.  And I was still allowing  myself to be perplexed by the whole business, with the two ounces of this and the half cup of that, because her housekeeping money each week did not cover all their needs.  I was trying to understand it when all I should have done was say 'no'. She could have cut down or borrowed from someone else.

# IN A PLACE OF DISCONNECTION

I was interfering.  I didn't realise at the time.  When I had coffee with her it was always made with half milk and half water, boiled up in a pan.  So one day I suggested to her that she make it with hot water and a dash like everybody else.  Then I started in on a homily.  That if - instead of things like mince and spaghetti dishes in the week and the big roast at weekends - she had, like me, egg and chips in the week, then the treat on Sunday could be the 'spag bog.'  She listened about the coffee, the dinners and then just said, 'I can't live that frugally.'  I was trying to help her out of her mess that was not really my business to do, other than react in whatever way I chose.
I did something that was quite manipulative when her husband helped me move heavy furniture prior to my re-decorating a room.  I bought a cheap bottle of wine to say 'thank you'. They always had a bottle of wine at the weekends, so I reckoned that my gift would release money for groceries.

The next day I popped round  to get back something long overdue, and there, sticking out of her kitchen bin was that bottle already empty.  When I confronted her with what my scheme for them had been, she just said that they could drink a bottle of wine any old day of the week and it was none of my business.  Going back down her path, I got another shock.  There, piled up against the dustbin, was what looked like a clear out of a year's magazines.

The cuttings never came my way either.But to be so blatant about it!  Why not hide those magazines from me? Or was I so much not in her head that she had not remembered my asking?
Like the cotton and sanitary towel, there was an ongoing situation at this time of something being `borrowed `when tit was actually being used up because there was no question of it ever being  returned.  One of her sons went to cubs and each week she came round to 'borrow' the shoe polish.

# Pamela Pickton

Around this time I met her as she came home with some shopping and there in her arms were bunches of flowers. 'Oh,' she said having the grace to look a bit sheepish. 'Our sitting room is so dead without flowers. Only a few shillings in the market. What's a few shillings?'A tin of shoe polish, I wanted to say.

She could not live without flowers any more than she could live 'frugally', she told me. Then there were the frequent parcels of books delivered from a book catalogue, general knowledge for the children, gardening and art for the adults. One arrived when I was there collecting my spoonfuls of this and that. 'I have to have beautiful things around me,' she said.

I was tearing my hair by now, and then I saw that the nearby Catholic school, where her children went, were presenting an evening and a Friar would be speaking and answering questions on faith and education. I went, and at the end he spoke to individuals alone. I told him about this woman and about my dilemma, about wanting to be kind and Christian,

'Ah,' he said, 'Jesus Christ never allowed himself to be made a fool. And there are other kind people in the world she could turn to.'

I remembered this when she wanted me to baby-sit on a day that was really difficult for me. I even went knocking on my other friends' doors on her behalf. Manipulating again. When that failed, in desperation I asked her if there were no one else she could ask. 'There is nobody else I can ask,' she replied, with a strong emphasis on the `nobody`. Nobody else who would take it.

As the years went by, so the behaviour intensified. These were the days of the shortages you remember, the shortages of potatoes, of loo paper and sugar? She had the nerve to come in for sugar – in a sugar shortage! I said I could spare very little, and thought it not needed to be said that I wanted it back very soon.  I called on her that evening with one of her parcels of glossy books which I had taken in for her, and she was just assembling one of those puddings that are layers and layers of meringue, with raspberries and cream in between.And I thought she needed the sugar for her children's cereal!

'Oh,' she said looking abashed.  'Meringue always looks a lot doesn't it?  A little bit of sugar does go a long way.'

Her mother retired and came to live with her for good. My neighbour seemed more frenzied, more worried about the extra pennies to buy the mushrooms - the extra garnish, for every meal.

Was mother the clue to it all, I wondered - the wanting to impress her mother?  Certainly, over the years I had picked up a bit about her family and childhood.  How there had been one brother, who was highly favoured as the only son and a sister who was the bee's knees, being flamboyant and very attractive.  How my friend had felt nothing in comparison to them.  So was it just some overwhelming sense of low esteem, some need to compensate, prove herself, show her mother that she was well off, which drove her to have and get and live at such a lavish level?  I knew that she was not happy with her appearance for she had said she was angry with God for not giving her either decent shaped legs or a pretty face, or at least boobs that were not totally flat.
'The only time I have felt truly a woman,' she told me, 'was when I was pregnant,'So that was the reason for the five children, I thought.

That came back to me when, around this time, I went to a counsellor about it all.
'She wants a bit of you,' the counsellor said.
I was reasonably attractive and had big boobs.  Was she taking from me as a kind of making things fair?  It was

funny because I myself considered my boobs too big, not easy to buy bras for or to fit into modern fashions. I thought I'd show her that the grass is not always greener and confessed the misery of the big boobs.

'I know,' she said. 'They are too big. You ought to have a partial mastectomy.'

I felt like saying, 'Would you like me to give the bits to you?'

The abuse really did step up once her mother moved back. My eldest had left home by now; I had no husband and basically no one for me. What few friends and relatives I had lost patience with my tales of the neighbour, saying I should be firmer. To make ends meet I ran a catalogue of clothes and household goods, sometimes getting orders from others to boost my commission. My neighbour did have one other friend who called, the one who had offered hera lift to the dressmaking class. This woman was well off and had that confidence which comes with money. She was no victim, would not be asked for anything – in fact my neighbour would want to impress her. Maybe that was who she cooked all those lavish meals for, as well as mother? This friend saw the catalogue in my neighbour's house and came to me asking if she could order something. Not thinking, I agreed to do it, and for the neighbour to collect the payments from her friend and give them to me.

One week I met the friend going into next-door and said that I had not had any payments for some weeks. She swore she had paid regularly and my neighbour insisted she had brought the payments round to me. But there were no tickings-off on my records. I knew I had not received the payments, and paid the catalogue from my own money.

Somebody once told me that everyone has a monster inside them and it was other people who allow it to grow.

# IN A PLACE OF DISCONNECTION

My complicity had certainly allowed an enormous monster to grow in my neighbour.  She borrowed something to wear, I said I needed it soon; she went off on holiday for two weeks leaving me without it.  She `borrowed` a neighbour's tub of margarine out of her fridge while cat sitting for her, and then was in a panic when she saw the neighbour arriving home from holiday earlier than expected.  She was talking to me at the gate when she saw the car draw up and visibly panicked.  Another time, when we met in the street, she suddenly darted indoors because another neighbour appeared.  'I have done some shopping for her and I've spent her change,' she explained as she went, and I wondered what she had been planning on doing about it.  Try to avoid the woman until she managed to scrape the cash from somewhere?  Or hope the woman would forget?

One day, I was so desperate for money myself, that I went to ask her for the ten pounds I had lent to her the week previously.  She had not expected me to need it so soon, did not have ten pounds, and said she supposed she would have to ask her husband.  Then she said me, 'can I say that it's not me paying back, but you borrowing?'

I could almost feel the time bomb that was ticking next door; the house bursting now that her mother was back, the budget bursting with trying to please mother or compensate for the boobs, or both.  It exploded.
The biggest borrow of all time.
My last child had left home and her eldest was planning on doing the same.  He was getting married.  Could the young couple move in with me, as there were so many of them and few of us?  Just for a little while, until they found somewhere. When I mumbled something about rent, she said that was absurd, that it was only like having a member of your own family to stay and that's what neighbours are for.

# Pamela Pickton

So son and girlfriend moved in with me, but the wedding did not take place and he stayed on.

'You should be more generous,' she said. 'He's had a shock. I've moved one of the younger ones into his room now. In fact I've spread them all out a bit, we`ve been so cramped. You must take Mother in too.'

That woman would bamboozle your month's salary out of your hand and convince you it was your Christian duty.

With those two in the house it became an extension of next door with the rest of the family in and out to visit. By now I was too exhausted to resist and the rest followed easily. The jilted boy went and the second moved away. The third was no longer of an age to bring in Family Allowance. With this source of income gone and I suppose her debts catching up with them, their house was to be repossessed. They were all to move in with me.

You do that for friends.

'We'll get back on our feet,' she said.

Well, they did not get back on their feet. They still have the weekend roasts, and the meringue fairy castles, and the wine. I could hardly bear it when I crept into the kitchen to cook my scraps.

'Why don't you get a gas ring put in your room, if you've going to be so unsociable?' she said.

'In fact there's a hand basin in that little back room, isn't there? Move in there. We can't be expected to feed you, how could we afford another mouth? Your house? Well that's there anyway. Why would you have it all to yourself? What a wicked waste.'

Nobody comes to visit me anymore. She is rude to them at the door. I think they've given up on me – think I'm mad or something. My children are both married and living hundreds of miles away. They do keep in touch but I don't see them. One was quite bitter on the phone recently.

# IN A PLACE OF DISCONNECTION

'You realise they are sitting tenants, Mother. They'll get your house in the end.'
So I have lost for my children their ultimate inheritance.

I had a bit of a turn recently, though as I don't get out much I didn't go to see a doctor. I've been a bit slow on my feet since then and shaky. I don't feel like going out much today. I'll just sit in my little room with its hand basin and gas ring. I have no pleasures now, what small income I have goes on the mortgage and overheads.

I just went down to them downstairs. I was about to make a cup of tea and found I had no sugar. So I just took my cup – it just happened to be in my hand – and went down to ask for a cup of sugar.

'Get you own,' she said.

# Pamela Pickton

STRIPES

'No, no satin, Madam.'
She flaps behind the counter like a frightened bird.
'Jersey? No I`m afraid not.'
Fluttery movements, feathery hair.
'... There`s some nice striped cottons.'

Pulling rolls of material out, pecking at the shelves; yes,
that`s it, trying to find a shred of gossamer for a nest.
'Plain? Well, of course there`s not much call for plain
these days.' Pursing her lips primly, reinforced by my
being so out of touch.

'Stripes are nice and fesh. Always look clean.'
Who says I want to look clean ?
'Evening dress? Oh, I see, well, let's have a look.'
A nervous mouse perhaps: the slight tremble, pushing the
spectacles up. Wispy curls like
whiskers. A nice story book mouse. Oh so eager to
please.
But I am the difficult customer.
Like a giant patchwork quilt, the materials are spilling over
the counter.
'Ginghams for curtains and denim for children's
overalls. Oh, dear, really only linens
here and haberdashery. Summer dress stuff, maternity
tops, a bit of heavy woollens for those
who can tailor. You know the sort of thing…
'Got a bit of lurex, remnant from the sale. Not enough
for you really. Brown and gold. Stripes.`
'I don`t want stripes,' I'm muttering now. I hope she
hasn`t heard me.
But, oh, all I want is something gorgeous. Something
different. You see, I just got a phone call. After five years,
he`s home from America. And coming round tonight.
Nothing very exciting to wear, but had a sudden thought.
Pop to the nearest shop and get a bit of stuff. Something
zany. Run it up quick. Just a shift, wouldn`t take long.

# IN A PLACE OF DISCONNECTION

Hold it all together with my chain belt.  No time to go far.
The flat, my hair, the meal to fix. Just thought I could pick
up something local.  Upholstery stuff even, brocade.
Something heavy and embossed would hang well.  I
knew you couldn`t expect much from these little shops,
but …!

  'Seersucker stripes  are quite pretty.'

  'I don't want to look pretty, I want to look seductive.'

  'Candy stripes are fresh.'

  'But not very sexy.'

  'Stripes are always clean.'

  I'd rather look debauched, but I won't tell her that.  I
just try to explain what I do want

  ' Black silk with cerise flowers you really wanted?

  'Oh, no dear. Only a little shop. There`s a nice pale blue
cotton with dark violets..'

Don't tell me.

'… arranged in stripes.'

I finger the baby gingham she offers me, looking wildly at
the walls.

Regency, grey and pink stripes.

She has grey and brown striped hair and stripes on her
face.

Spots and dainty polka dots dance in my eyes and I see
fresh yellow and white stripes

blowing on the kitchen curtain breeze.

Clean stripes, clean blue and white tiles in bands, stand
guard over our kitchen hygiene.

And stiff red stripes on my mother`s apron, tied round my
waist and reaching to the floor, as I

rolled and re-rolled the leather pastry, anchored me in my
unwilling domesticity.

  'I don't want stripes.'

I scream, she cringes.

 'I don't want cotton or gingham or daisy prints.'

She shrinks away.

  'Well, madam, I don't know what to do for you.'

  'Something exotic. My old flame is coming.'

# Pamela Pickton

'Shocking pink,madam? I`m sure we have some somewhere.'

'I don`t want pink, or blue or yellow...'

I'm tearing my hair.

'.. they`re the colours of innocence.'

`Well, really, I don't know what to say. `

'I'd rather look wicked.'

'Let`s see. We may still have some blackout stuff downstairs.'

'I've got to make this up in half an hour.'

'Some pretty organdie here..'

'Too difficult. I don't sew well. Something easy, something heavy, just drop into a shift.'

'Let me get the stepladder.  Look, some cotton velvet..'

'Oh?'

'Dusty pink. Powder blue.'

'No.'

Rummaging in the bottom drawer..'You said you wanted black?'

'Show me.'

Black.

With white stripes.

Stripes. More stripes. Good girl stripes. Nurse`s uniforms.

Chalk thin stripes on teacher`s dark blouse.

Cool green or pristine blue on virgin white.

There are parallel lines between her teeth. She still smiles after all this.  But her hands are
pressed together in symmetrical prayer.

I look down to her sacrifice of thin and thick stripes before me, and my eyes zig-zag again.

I close them and see, not the lines, but a blaze of colour.

A magenta of peony.

Is it the dress of my dreams?  No, I`ve seen it somewhere.

My heart is pounding now with a sense of coming home.

Somewhere there is a piece of material she is hiding from me.

The bags!

# IN A PLACE OF DISCONNECTION

The shop's paper bags, hanging on a hook. Deep pink
with a black rose in the middle, for
the shop is called ' Rose.'
   Perhaps she is called Rose too, and at night takes off
        her spectacles and puts a rose behind
her ear, and dances in chiffon bought elsewhere.
   'How much are the bags?'
   'I beg your pardon, madam?'
   'I`d like to buy some of your pink paper bags.'
   'Well, I don't know, I suppose so, madam. I don't see
        why not.'
   'How many would it take if I ripped them down the sides
        and glued them to a belt, to make
a sort of skirt?  Not joined or anything. Just loose.
        Hawaii.'
Oh, dear, what a suspicious look. Now she is pulling the
        whole lot off the wall. Just wants to
get rid of me now. I can't blame her.
   'I'm sorry we couldn't satisfy you madam. Please take
        these with our compliments.'
   'Thank you,' and I retreat with only one glance back at
the festive jubilee array in the window: striped towels,
striped pillow cases, I stride out into the splash of
clashing colours, the haphazard interweaving of people,
and the satin ripple of traffic of my world.
At least it will be easy to make up.
And if it tears during the evening....
Well.....

# Pamela Pickton

THE HOURS

Queenie Dalloway had to do it all herself. There was nobody else.

What a name. She had never forgiven her mother. You would have thought, with a surname like that, there were many more appropriate choices, even the most obvious one; but it was often so. She had not been born in England, and when somebody English has a baby while living abroad, they often get it wrong, and middle class people end up with names frowned on at home. It was not only the tone, the class connotations, that these parents got wrong, nowadays giving their children names like Tracey or Sharon, but often they were names out of time as well. Her daughter's friend, of her generation and born in Hong Kong, had been named Ken and his brother Stanley.

She loved her surname and could that be, she sometimes wondered, why she had not married, in spite of becoming pregnant? Some women do keep their names, she knew that, but not so much in the sixties. The fact that he was called Pratt might have had something to do with it, she sometimes laughingly admitted to friends. Or even the fact that he turned out to be something that rhymed with his name.

Of course her name being what it was she had early become a Woolf reader. But it was only on reading The Hours, Michael Cunningham's recent work based on the book of her namesake, that something had struck her. For she had read it soon after sending out the invitations for this party today.

Mrs. Dalloway decided to buy the flowers herself! Goodness me, how big. And when she was reading of that day spent by the more modern namesake, she remembered yet another book written somewhere

# IN A PLACE OF DISCONNECTION

between the Woolf and the Cunningham. In that, a novel by Margaret Drabble, the last chapter was the day of a party. And what did the hostess do that day? She went out to buy a tree! A small tree it is true: a pretty tree, a garden tree. While reading that when she was younger, Queenie had been amazed that anyone who had a party that evening should spend time strolling around a garden centre, talking about this and that to the son who had gone with her to buy it.

Surely she had other things to attend to, she had thought. And then, at the end of that chapter, at the end of that book, how was the hostess left? What was the end of the story of that woman and her life? Why, she was searching through her wardrobe for something to wear to her party. One dress had the hem hanging down. Others had broken zips or stains or buttons off or were torn or no longer fitted. Readers left the author`s heroine, with the party about to start, sitting on her bed going though all these possible outfits and wondering what to do.

Maybe it is me, she had thought at the time, envying the luxury of mind in being able to get up on the day that you were throwing a party in your house and think, oh what shall we do today? I know, let`s go out and buy a tree to make the garden look nice for the do. Then, to have left what to wear to the very last minute!

She envied such a relaxed state of mind; for surely it would all turn out. Surely at least one of the garments would be fixable. Yet she knew that she could never be like that, she was the sort who planned and prepared way ahead for all events and for their eventualities. She was not a relaxed person, and when she once told a friend of that character in a book who, it seemed, had given no prior thought as to what to wear for her party, that friend replied that she herself knew a couple of women who would be just the same.

# Pamela Pickton

` They would just wear anything, ` the friend told her. `
Even if they had to resort to track suit bottoms and a
jumper that did not go.

 Such women must be rare, Queenie had thought to
herself, and throughout the lead up to this her own party,
the newest Mrs. Dalloway  was on her mind for she was
reading the book. How could anyone be so relaxed – be
out and about – when they were giving a party that very
evening? The story of Laura Brown in The Hours, is also
the story of one day. Laura too has a party at the end of
that day, albeit a family birthday party with only her
husband and child. But as well as making two birthday
cakes ( because one is a failure), wrapping presents,
getting ready house,  meal, table, and self; as well as
looking after a child and starting as she does with a late
rising through being pregnant and depressed, she still
manages a lengthy trip out on her own to get away from it
all. How do other people fit in so much Queenie worried
as she read the book and planned for her own party.

   Then with the passing days came the memory of that
book written in the sixties. That one had always been at
the back of her mind; she had never gotten over the
picture of that woman sitting on her bed, the party about
to begin, examining, seemingly without hope or plan, her
hopeless garments. When she finished the Cunningham
she considered re reading the original Mrs. Dalloway. And
even as she hunted the old copy in her bookshelves, a
forgotten detail came back to her even before she opened
the pages, before she even located the book. Of course.
The first Dalloway - Clarissa - too had gone to her closet
and found that the dress - presumably the only possible
dress, or at least the one she intended to wear - was torn.
It was only for the first time now, thirty or more years on,
that she had ever seen the parallel between the Dalloway
party and that of the heroine  in Margaret Drabble`s
novel. Was that where Miss Drabble had got the idea?

# IN A PLACE OF DISCONNECTION

Strange the parts of a book you remember, even when you recall little else of it. She could not have told anyone the title of that Drabble book nor what it was about. She realised now that, with a lifetime of reading behind her, she could have listed relatively few. Strange how, beginning with poems and stories of childhood, even bits from comics, then the reading from adulthood until her fifties, that she remembered so little. If asked she may have remembered more; but what was interesting was the fact that her head was filled most of the time with a few snippets and quotations.

Maybe everyone is like that she thought now, and maybe the few lines which stick in our heads are what would tell most about us – almost bypass many years of the analyst`s couch.

Mrs. Dalloway did at least set to and mend her dress herself; but as with the flowers you felt she was being supremely good. She bought the flowers herself, she mended the dress herself : she would not bother the servants. But the point was that there were servants to whom she could, if need be, delegate both tasks.

Queenie Dalloway`s finances do not run to caterers and she has no servants to clean her silver. She has no silver and is using some throw away plates and napkins and even forks. This is a party for her daughter who had just published her first book. The girl insisted on a party, and Queenie agreed albeit asking her daughter to accept that it would not be a lavish affair and that in fact close friends would be asked to contribute dishes of food.

Am I in fact mean she asked herself now beginning to pull frozen dishes from her freezer. She is not wealthy it is true but she had often noted poorer friends who were more hospitable: would butter and make a delicacy of their last slice of bread as it were. Was it something to do with not wanting to give, not wanting to feed? She remembered the cow who refuses to give the king some butter for his bread.

It was interesting too how differently one`s friends received such news. `A party?` one had looked bright, then, ` oh, bring our own food,` she had smirked . Others had said what a good idea I often do the same myself, I`ll bring you a dish of my party special.`

Nevertheless, she has been involved in cooking for some weeks. Since the invitations went out, her days have been packed with the cleaning then tidying of the house and garden, then creating dishes she could freeze. Her clothes she sorted out very early on in her ` Party Calendar `, gingerly hand - washing something which she knew should really go to the Dry Cleaners. There would be no flowers. She had not thought about that until today when the recent reading and the nature of the day ahead of her had brought back the opening line of those two stories.

Today then, this day of her party, she rises early, showers and blow dries her hair then puts on a track suit which will do until nearer the time. The basic daily tidying of the house, making her bed, putting away last bits of drying washing, hiding today`s post to sort another day, sees the clock tick away an hour as she ends those preparations with laying out to the last pin all the cosmetic and baubles she will need for her final dressing. Then, the food out of the freezer, she sets to preparing the vegetables bought yesterday, and assembling them into different salads.

The minutes tick by the hours of the morning. Cutting and preparing those vegetables, polishing furniture, setting out the table with the bowls for nibbles, the arranging of cheeses on a board, are all interrupted by telephone calls. Could I bring so and so ..? Is it all right if I come a bit early, or a bit late, because of this or that? Would she

mind if Linda came an hour late  (even thought Linda was
bringing  some major dishes .)

She works through, swallowing a banana and some dried
fruit and nuts for lunch to save on washing up. There is
furniture to be moved, pushed back against walls, chairs
to be brought in from shed or down from attic. Fred calls.
He was to be bringing all the French bread. He can`t do it.
He will now only be able to come half way through. She
calls her best friend Susan. Can Susan bring the bread?
Susan says yes but calls back half an hour later to say
that her shop is out of it. Queenie will have to buy the
bread herself. No amble for her though, no stroll as with
the flowers and the tree. Into car, still with her house
shoes still on, round to her nearest small supermarket
which makes the bread there so that they never run out.
Back in half an hour. Then what seemed like another half
hour to unload the loaves from the car.

Is her oven ready for the last minute warming of brought
quiches and things?  No, her oven is full, as usual, of
baking trays and tins. She remembers how, for her last
party, and although asked not to, many of her friends
brought vegetarian dishes or curries which had needed
heating or even cooking.  Oh, she still has not cleared
enough space on tables and kitchen work surface for the
drinks the water, the mixers, the bowl of ice....better
check there is enough of that in the freezer, but of course
she did that days ago.  Has she washed the jugs?  No.
Glasses to polish and large plates and bowls for serving
( people will bring food in plastic tubs) were rooted out or
borrowed yesterday.

At the last minute, she would start tipping out nibbles. Or
perhaps half an hour before – for she remembers those
who have already said they would turn up early. There
were bound to be several who would turn up far too soon.
Always in her life were those who had got it wrong or
whose bus had brought them quicker than they thought;

# Pamela Pickton

and they sat and talked as she prepared food or had to be left with a book of the television while she finished dressing. How she hated that, being caught it seemed to her with her knickers down. For so it was, for her, to be opening the door when she had not made up her face.

Plagued all day with her nervous IBS, she holds her breath every time she dashes to the loo, lest there be an inopportune knock on the door.

Then Josie calls to say they have been ill all week and have only just remembered the party and that they had promised desserts. Josie loves cooking and had promised four different puddings. While commiserating with the illness, Queenie asks herself whether she should buy cheeseakes and things herself. Putting the phone down and looking at the clock, she begins dialling. Watching the clock tick many minutes which seem like many hours, she dials many numbers until she finds people who are both in and who can promise to bring one sweet something.

She begins to wonder if she does indeed have enough bread, thinking how much went last time, racks her brain again and scours the cupboards and fridge. She has those miserable things called bread sticks and half a cut loaf to make toast. What the hell – who needs bread? Already here is salmon and ham and salad and cheese and crackers. Coronation chicken and quiches, rice and pasta salads will be coming. She hopes.

In the course of the day one friend does call her saying she can`t come giving some feeble excuse but sounding black .Only half an hour later does Queenie wonder if this friend is in fact her Richard Brown - the friend in one of the other books who is about to commit suicide. Well, if she had servants and caterers she would go to their aid; and anyway what point if they had made up their mind to

# IN A PLACE OF DISCONNECTION

tip themselves out of  a window, one way or another, in spite of friendly administrations?

Is kindness, is charity, a luxury she asks herself, and explores again the age old question of altruism. If it is true, she thinks, that we do nothing without some self interest,  then that is borne out by the fact that I am not prepared to play lady bountiful when I am too busy.

Even then though, as she dusts a chest which had been somehow missed, she has a new thought on that old debate. Surely she asks herself, if I were in need, would I really care how pure were the motives of my helpers – as long as I got the help?

At that time when Margaret Drabble`s heroine is sorting through her clothes, Queenie is putting on the ear rings placed ready last night when she remembers that none of the white wine is in the fridge  to cool and that there is probably no room. Would it be too soon to take the salad out?

And as the first knock on the door comes she looks at the hall table, bare except for a few photographs. No flowers.

It is her daughter. She can see her shape through the glass of the front door. And - does she, is she - holding an armful of flowers?

(Oh, drat, Queenie thinks miserably, knowingly ungrateful. Now she will have to find vases. Do arranging.)

` Here I am , ` says her daughter. ` Is everything ready?`

` Of course it is, darling.

`And thank you for the flowers.`

# Pamela Pickton

FAMILY   MONOLOGUES

THE FATHER

Aren't you driving a bit fast, Dad? Sit still, Amy, don't jump on my tummy. You know Mummy has a little baby in there, a baby brother or sister for you. Look out of the window, Granddad will soon get us home.  No need to rush, Dad. There's plenty of time. We've had a lovely day, a lovely day at the seaside haven't we Amy?  Isn't it kind of Granddad to take us out? Ray wont be home 'til seven and I've left a salad all ready. No, you can't go and sit in the front with Nanny.  Look at all the cars. There, Nanny has given you another sweetie. Now sit still! Ooh, Dad, I thought we were going into that bus then. Ouch, now she's fallen on me. Yes, she's hurt  her head. Some people are getting seat belts now, you know. Don't cry, darling, you should not have been standing up like that. But we are going a bit fast, don't you think so, Mum? Oh, Dad, do be careful. I told you there's no hurry. Oh, I know Amy said she wanted to go to the loo, but she's forgotten about it now and anyway we could stop somewhere surely, there's no need to kill us all. Christ, I thought we were going  over then, you took that corner so sharp. Has he gone daft, Mum? Why doesn't he take any notice of me? Look we're doing ninety. Stop it! Can't you hear me? Amy's crying and you'll start the baby coming in a minute. You know I haven't got long to go. What? The car's making so much noise I can't hear you. Cancer? Whatever are you talking about? Six months? You? No! Stop it, can't you hear me? That wall, that wall, turn Dad, turn. The baby, Dad, The baby. You don't care? We all spoilt your life? Already had more than you ever had? Well, you can't take us all with you. Dad? You can't mean that? Turn the wheel! Please. Oh, God.

# IN A PLACE OF DISCONNECTION

FAMILY MONOLOGUES CONTINUED

THE MOTHER

THEN . My mother, draining me, always asking more. Quiet, moaning, bullying, always one more thing, never enough. Just do this for me. Mind your little brother for me. Look after the whole house while I go away for a break.

NOW. it`s just cut my hair for me, turn up my coat, decorate my room, dig my garden. Meet me in the shops, have coffee with me, tea, lunch. Take me to the park; bring a picnic, a friend for me, a car for me to ride in. Lend me your dress your jewellery your house your children to take out and show off. Give me a lift, a theatre trip, a stay with you. Find me a job, a friend, a new flat.

My mother. It was always the same message to me: `don't worry me, don't want anything, don't trouble me by being miserable.   Don't bother me by being anything. Don't be.`

Now, I say yes Mother no Mother what next Mother, anything but the nagging, the whining, the crying on the phone: ` What a dreary life I have, never had anything, never go anywhere nobody cares about me.`

Now the final attack! My face at the window of my brother`s car white, staring, haunted, though no one could save me even if they saw me, for no laws are being broken. No laws are involved only the vicious binding unwritten laws of the umbilical cord. My face at the window and sick gorge rises in me as the car moves off.

  I have been summoned to my mother for the last time - `it was your mother`s last wish, `- and I have been fetched to lay her out.

# Pamela Pickton

FAMILY MONOLOGUES CONTINUED

THE CHILD

A lazy afternoon, the children half watching television, Tony running his cars up and down over the cushions, Sophie lying on her tummy colouring with felt pens, Mark who has been doing his homework, now curled up with a comic. I have been helping him with his geometry and he has left his exercise book and pencil case next to me on the sofa where I sit sewing. We often enjoy a relaxed day like this when Bob has to work on a Saturday. The baby is crawling all over me, I must be careful with the needles. Now, she has rolled onto the floor and pulled herself up against the sofa. Oh, no, Mark has left his pencil case undone and she has got everything out. Let me hide that sharp compass quick. She is jut on the point of walking, our lovely Emma. I carry her with me under my arm to make a cup of tea. I am used to tucking babies under one arm, while the other hand  pours the hot water. Better than leaving her crawling where I can`t see her. The children are playing a boxed game now. I put my favourite music on. Sophie runs upstairs crying about something not being fair. Tony throws the game board up in the air and Mark switches the television back on. The baby falls on the scissors as Sophie comes back in the room.

If I sit her up on the sofa as she was, buttons all around her, things might go on the same.
It was such a silly little moment.

# IN A PLACE OF DISCONNECTION

THERE`S SOMETHING OUTSIDE

The main thing was not to let the children see she was afraid. She must carry on as usual, in a minute get their tea. Go to the kitchen, with that big window. Just as though there was no danger outside, no prowler at their gate. To think we are not safe even in our own home, Mary thought. They talked of an English man's home, but what castle would withstand an enemy - or an act of God?

While she gave them tea she would have to laugh with them. She made herself a strong coffee and drank it quickly trying, with everything she did, not to look at the window. Even putting water in the kettle she turned her head away, judging everything by feel. She swallowed the coffee as though hoping she was drinking in strength. Then, taking a deep breath, she walked into the living room where the children were playing. She smiled at her two little girls and the boy who had come to play, even forced a laugh when Toby hurtled across the room, rolly-pollying at her feet.

But she could not face it all, not yet. A far distant but unmistakeable tremor sent her looking around in desperation. She grabbed a magazine, hoping they would think that was why she had come in, and sought secrecy by covering her face with it, hoping it would mask her gasps of fear. Then, for a time, she sat on the stairs, clutching her shoulders and rocking, rocking. Oh, if only they could hide.

It made it worse having her friend`s child to look after. With her own, she might not have felt quite so much pressure to keep an icy exterior of being in control. She could hardly scream in front of a visitor. Then a new fear grasped her. Supposing her friend was late home and rang Mary to bring Toby to her? Then she would actually have to go outside. But now she must go to the children and distract them for the bangs were nearer now, like gunfire. They might be getting scared. The news had been given out earlier that day of a terror at large, but Mary had hoped the enemy might not come this close.

Life was cruel. She remembered her ski-loving friends and that fragile cabin. Why had the avalanche had to choose there? Well, nobody could help Mary either, but at least she could make it as easy as possible for her children. And so she sat with them on the floor and played Happy Families. And she did her best to join in though she had to force her lips to smile, her voice to laugh. But all the time inside there was this sinking turning over thud, at the fire crackers, the faint pistol pop pops, coming nearer.

Mandy accused Toby of cheating and he pulled her hair. Mary had to go through the motions of telling them off but she did it in a flat mechanical voice. What did it all matter anyway? She looked at the children`s soft arms and the long lashes against sweet cheeks. She was trying in vain to push away a vision of their whole bodies, face and all, covered by blankets.

The fear would not let her keep still and she fidgeted as she played, unable to concentrate even at a surface level. Her head was sick and spinning and there was no room for other thoughts so, as soon as she could, she escaped. Her agitation took her to the kitchen because she had to move, had to do something. The walking was really an attempt to run from fear, when what she really wanted was to get up and run from herself - not be herself with this all-consuming terror. Mary felt as you feel when you drop something precious and catch it just in time, but you are left with a lurching sickness and an after- pain of shock that shoots to your fingers and toes.

She was still not looking out of the window and although the winter afternoon was coming to an end, she had not

# IN A PLACE OF DISCONNECTION

dared to get close enough to draw the curtains here or anywhere else in the house. Now, she decided to force herself to pull down the kitchen blind, but getting even half way near enough was too awful. What had been only a remote patter was now a thud, a pad. This thing at large was it already so close?

She turned her back to the window and began making the tea. When she was like this, obsession filled her head, everything around her a brightly lit unreal world. She was so shut up, alone with her darkness, that everything else was a dream and the hands that made the meal did not seem to belong to her. She had to tell them to pick up a knife force them to spread butter, and when she walked to the cupboard for biscuits it was as though she were floating. And it was as she turned from the cupboard, clutching the cylindrical cellophane-wrapped object and wondering what it was and what she was meant to be doing, that she heard herself scream. Claire had opened the kitchen door. It was agape. The child was standing there, looking out.

In the space of no time, Mary banged the door shut, slapped the child fiercely, fixed all the keys and bolts, and jerked down the small door blind. Then she turned to the crying child feeling her own face hot and tight. She hugged Claire, kissed her, told her she was sorry. It was all right. It was just that it was getting a bit late and cold. She was worried about them all catching chills, she had not meant to make such a fuss. She gave Claire a heap of sweets to share out and called out that tea would not be long. Now she hated herself and the tears ran down her face. She ran round the house to hide them from the children, forcing herself to close all the curtains and willing the tears to go away. When she dragged herself back to the kitchen, Mandy was there and, as Mary cooked sausages and beans, she was at her elbow talking in that way children do that is too much when your head is full to bursting.

# Pamela Pickton

'One of my friends at school knew someone who got killed with this…'

'Don't be silly, of course you can`t get killed.'

Mary was snapping now and at the end of her tether. Hadn`t she heard of enough incidents herself, but the child was making her focus on what she was trying to push away.

Yet again she had to will herself not to scream. Instead she fetched the children and sat them on kitchen stools. She must chatter brightly. The danger would either pass or would get them. But at least they must not know, must be happy until their last minute. The shock of the noise outside was so great that she spilled the milk she was pouring into mugs. The horror was really close now, it could happen any time. With clenched fists she faced it. In seconds they could all be dead.

Calmly she answered their questions about what was going on outside, scarcely believing the coolness of her own voice. She knew all the technical sensible facts and was pleased to see they were persuaded, unafraid, even quite excited by it all.  Strange really, Mary thought, that you could know the scientific truths yet still be terrified. But then you could not ignore that there was a possibility, no expert could deny it. A chance in a million, a billion, a trillion - maybe, but somebody had to be that one statistic.

The moment was here and the panic inside her was fierce. She had to force herself to sit tight on her stool and make her hands help cut toast, pass ketchup.  Mary was so busy spreading jam and refilling mugs that at first she did not realise the peak of the crisis had passed, the moment of real danger. She forced herself to get up and make more strong coffee.

The thunderstorm was over.

# IN A PLACE OF DISCONNECTION

## THE OPEN WINDOW

Going to the window, she drew back the curtains.

And  just as when you try to savour something in your mouth, just as then you cannot taste it – perhaps it has been too much anticipated, this chocolate, this cream cake – and too much you want to make it last, this taste you cannot have very often, and you concentrate so hard that you cannot realise the taste; just as also you might stare at a beloved face about to depart – what is it you love about it, how can you imprint it on your memory, to remember it when apart – and so you stare and try to experience the 'here and now' which is so small because so fleeting  - and how can five minutes of chocolate in the mouth sink into consciousness which has been waiting for it for five months, any more than you can enjoy the face when a future without it lies ahead?   So the outside world had no impact, meant nothing, she felt nothing. So much out there had happened, was remembered, hated, but the return to the world had been too intently awaited and the moment fell flat.

But this was still a great event. She looked, not too closely, not enjoying what she saw, but pleased with this tremendous effort. What was it they had said at school? That to add one to nought is to add infinity? Because to add anything to nothing is as big a step as adding any number. So, after all these months, for her to get out of a chair, open her curtains and look out on the street, was as if she had gone to the ends of the earth.

How many months was it? She didn't really know. It is strange the way time passes. She had always pitied prisoners but now she could see that twenty years could pass as one eternal day of breakfast, a few odd jobs, lunch, a little read, tea, a bath, the radio, a cup of cocoa, and bed. You can fill your time, tell yourself you really do need to wash that one sweater slowly, you are not just filling in time because it must be done gently. And so, carefully, you do a neat darn in the time it would take a teenager to shower, blow dry hair, paint nails, make up her face, dress, and run out of the door. You are heavy. Legs drag and arms are slow. Your eyes are hazy and you can hardly see. After nights of relentless thinking, a nagging thread that wont be left taking you into a tangle of knots, round and round and never coming to an end; after the tossing and pain and clenching of fists, of staring into the dark, so you come to day with woolly brain and filmed eyes.

She had felt like this before, from time to time recurring. Though not so badly. She should have known, been prepared. Then, she had got low, had that bad flu and when she went back to work found her job had gone. She was not wanted anymore. She had walked the streets in a daze, the glaring shops filled with grinning successful people, happy job takers. She alone lost, different, cut off from this alien world.

Her confidence shaken she could not look for a job straightaway. A rest at home might pick her up. But then. The neighbour rushing to tell her. Why is it people love to share bad news? She always kept such things to herself, so that two years later a mutual friend might say what about 'old so and so' haven't seen them lately and she would have to say. Dead. Other people seemed to revel, gloat, as if they thought this way they faced the bogeyman and frightened him away. So there the woman was anyway, from the flat upstairs, bra strap showing, big teeth and tapping out her ash. Didn't she know that Maggie downstairs had died? 'Well of course I hadn't seen her around last week or two...in hospital of course...yes. Cancer...only thirty-nine...didn't even look ill to me...makes you think, doesn't it, who`s turn next? Well, this won't buy the baby a new pair of drawers will it ducks? Ta Ta'

# IN A PLACE OF DISCONNECTION

Thirty-nine. She was thirty-five herself. You never knew. Any day. You might wake up to find a lump, or walking round the supermarket, go out like a light, ambulance man carrying the blanket covered stretcher. Insignificant among the trolleys, that's it, over. So what, who was she anyhow?

The obsession had grown fast 'til it pervaded everything, everyone she looked at. Why are they smiling when one day, any day, finished? Underground next week? Have a coffee, coffee, coffee – coff, coff, coffin, coffin. Like some cream? How could they mouth the sound cream? Cream – cremate, cremated, cremation. Soon she could hardly get up in the morning, what point in the day? No point in anything. She was afraid to shut her eyes at night in case she died in her sleep.

The worst thing was the shops. The crowd of non-caring smilers, stressing her isolation, what matter to them if she died suddenly, got run over? Her mind so death orientated she gravitated to all those news items about disaster as if she had to make herself know the worst. She seemed to be on some sort of wavelength that found nothing but these headlines, every tiny one. Man drops dead in street. Mother of twenty has sudden fatal heart attack. Never a day`s illness say family of youth who fell, forever, at school sports.

There seemed to be nothing else. This was all life was. And any time it could be her. She began to tremble when she went out shopping. Somehow the panic, the certainty of imminent death, did not come over her so much at home. Perhaps it was the anonymity in the shops, no identification, no phone, no lifeline to a doctor. Soon she felt sick at the very thought of going out and once there had to rush straight back. And so she did not go out anymore. She told her neighbour that she had a bad back and although the woman did look a bit suspicious, she agreed to bring some shopping in.

# Pamela Pickton

But even indoors things got worse. In the end she could not bear to read or listen to the radio, lest just one word led her back to fear. The lack of exercise together with constant tension  caused aches and pains that convinced her she was dying anyway. But sometimes she wondered if she could be mad, for other people seemed to enjoy life. She often heard shouts and laughter outside; perhaps she was wicked because she did not, as others did, accept the human lot and enjoy what there was.

Everything was black, was nothingness. She hated living but was terrified of killing herself. There was nowhere to go. It was like a brick wall, a dead end block in her mind. Death was terrible and life was only thoughts of death. Nor could she go for help, for how could she inflict this misery on someone else? And something else - rebellion? - made her not want to go somewhere where she would be persuaded not to mind what she did mind.

Rebellion. Was this something new? For something in her had began to stir. This could not be how it was meant to be, or why was there life at all? Others were not so haunted - was it just her way of looking at things? Something in her had not died, though her hair was lank and her skin dead. Something like life still kicked in her, for when she did put the radio on a certain song reminded her of how she had always wanted to join a choir. An obstinate craving still nagged for more - more people, more action, all the experience she could seize.

If her desire to live and be had survived this withdrawal from life, could this not be a sign of some spark within her that would survive the actual death of the body? In any case, it must make more sense to live fully, if only for forty years, than live like this. But still she trembled. The thought of walking out of that door, of braving the shops, of seeking a job, made her sick. One thing at a time. If she could only walk to the gate every day for a week, that would be a start.

# IN A PLACE OF DISCONNECTION

All morning she sat in her chair, gripping the arms, clutching at them as she tried to make the huge effort of that initial step. The curtains had been shut for so long. She heaved herself up. Sick, not at all hopeful, but convinced she must try something even if it were no good. If only she could open those curtains who knew what other doors would open for her?

In the depths of an indescribable horror, beyond the point of actual thoughts or feelings, just impossibly awful - perhaps the darkness before the dawn - she moved to the window and drew back the curtains.

# Pamela Pickton

CRIME AND PUNISHMENT

The man hanged at dawn was still hanging at noon, and in the heat of the midday sun, the traveller could not disregard the groans. So he ordered his servant to whip the thirsty horse to halt and leant out of his carriage.

'My good man, I hear that you suffer. Hangmen are scoundrels  themselves, and are at no pains to make the despatch fast.'

The hanged man heard but could not answer. He tried but, from delirium, his thoughts reached the traveller`s ears as gibberish. And still his legs kicked out on their own as if they had not given up hope of finding a foothold. A hold on life.

The traveller, small and squat below, noted the red mouthing face.
'I do not know why you make such ado,' he mopped his own brow with silken kerchief.    'You only meet your just deserts.'
The rope felt tighter now and for a moment he felt it would soon be over, must be over soon. Almost he could wish this. But now he did begin to thrash his legs himself as if to break away and his screams came clear at last.

'It hurts you fool, it hurts.'
'Of course, what did you expect?  Did you never consider the consequences?'
'It hurts too much,' he was whimpering.
'Yes but, my good man, you are not the only one. Thousands have hanged before and worse.
You should be grateful you are not by now on the quartering table.'

Impatient, he walked back to his carriage and ordered his man to labour the horse so they might make up lost time. What did the man want? That he should hasten his end or perhaps cut him down and revive him, so risking his own captivity?

The audacity. The traveller was sure that, in payment for sin, he would not assail the ears of passers-by with such cries. It must sorely distress the ladies. And so he continued his journey. He who had locked up his witless brother and taken his inheritance, a crime not traced; and who beat his wife and nightly raped her – acts not considered to be crimes. He took a sip from his flask - the parched baked tongue already forgotten.

The bad man knew the traveller was right. Many hanged and many got worse. He had always known the risk. He had watched wretches swing, yet still had brought the same on himself.

The screams grew quieter on his lips though louder in his head. They stuck in his throat. And besides, nobody came

Of course the man was right. But the prisoner wished someone could have described the pain. It might have prevented........

What he really wanted, in the last flickers of consciousness, was to be cuddled and cry, 'Mummy, Mummy.'

The insane realms of pain. Had he not always been an orphan?

Stupid to have hoped the traveller might have held his hand to the end.

# Pamela Pickton

DECKCHAIR DAD

Man in a deckchair, what do you see?

See a man in a deckchair. He is reading a newspaper. And suddenly he is her Dad. And if you watch closely, he is not really looking at the paper. He is peering over it and watching the girls on the beach around him, the girls in bikinis.

There was this play she wanted to go and see. She had heard of it, a funny show with a famous comic actor in it. And the family usually went to a pantomime or something at Christmas anyway. Dad said he would go to it but on the day, when they got there, she found it was not that show at all. Dad just said, ' I don't like farces.'

She doesn't remember what it was called. Must have been some kind of revue, with all sorts of entertainers in it, jugglers, magicians or slapstick clowns. She hoped so because some of his children, were even younger than her. All she can remember is the line of girls dancing, seemingly forever. Dancing in front of them and right in front of the stage in front of their noses, kicking their legs high to every note of every tune, and showing the thin strip of material which covered their most private parts.

The man in the deckchair brings back those girls and her Dad looking at them as he does the girls on the beach. And it brings back how he looked at her. It began when she was about eleven and woke to feel him looking at her. Looking at her in her bed, with her covers kicked off and her nightie ridden up, maybe from fitful or nightmare filled sleep. She thought at first he was fatherly re-covering her to keep her warm, but before he replaced the bedding was a long time. She knew he was looking at her with the nightdress round her waist. And pretended to be asleep.

# IN A PLACE OF DISCONNECTION

Another time, he picked her up seemingly to play with her, in a daddily kind of way before she went to bed. She was in her nightdress and was confused because, you see, she was not a child who got cuddles or affection or even attention from either parent. He picked her up and swung her round and she knew when he stopped he was facing her bedroom mirror and that what he could see was her bottom half below his arms and with the nightie fallen away. And no knickers.

He began to take her swimming. It felt odd, just her out of a large family. They were a family of swimmers. That's what they did. Their only outing you might say. They lived near a seaside resort. Where men sat on the beach in deckchairs, and with newspapers.

But this was to the baths. Maybe it was because she was the oldest. It tended to be her who was invited to places out of their large family because she supposed she was amenable. It was nice to go swimming at first and, at first, good to feel she was getting all the attention. But as they walked there he put his arm round her and in the water he did the same. Arms round her shoulders – not Daddy holding little girl's hand – but as if she were his girlfriend.

When he came in to her room to kiss her goodnight in her nightie, those times, he hugged her pressing their two bodies all the way down - from chest to beginning of legs. People would know what she meant. And it did not feel right. She was not a kissed and cuddled child. And beside this felt like the sort of kissing you saw at the pictures, the sort of kiss films stars did. Men and ladies.

Another time she woke and found her dad was in her bed. And she pretended to be asleep.

# Pamela Pickton

CINDERELLA

My life is a dustbin. I am a dustbin. Dustbin they called me at school, when I ate up the greasy fritters and rubbery sausages rejected by the rich girls. Who would not be a dustbin for any old dry crust, when often there was no breakfast or even any tea at home?

I was the dustbin for others` cast off rags and worn out shoes. At Christmas I was the receptacle for broken toys. Later, there was warmth and comfort and food when I was taken to the place where many children go.

Then I became the dustbin for affection, grasping at any scraps of attention. Remnants perhaps of a failed marriage, some other woman`s leavings. I was an ever, open bin - always hopeful that the dust might be gold. Empty, empty, I waited to be filled, and filled I sometimes was, for the visitors to the bin left their visiting cards. Then, I was taken to the place where many girls go.

Now, I am full to bursting, waiting only to be emptied of all the trash I have collected and which has gone sour. Oh, I know all about rubbish bins for I have emptied many - swept round them, even searched through them for some madam's lost treasures. Dustbins are the only truth of people`s lives.

It would seem that people think they are magic: that when something is put in a dustbin it disappears. Do people think that dustmen and servants have no eyes or powers of deduction? All the sordid evidence of illegality or deceit, they don't go unnoticed. It can be like turning up a lovely shiny stone and finding the rotten crawling life underneath, searching through the contents of some respectable man`s bin.

My brain is a dustbin, as I read other people`s newspapers and listen to next door`s music coming

# IN A PLACE OF DISCONNECTION

through the wall. Second hand experiences from all my idle madams are all that I am worth. If my family had been kind – never mind wealthy – I might have gone on in education. Now, all the tons of rubbish and the hot ashes of despair have deadened my mind; I would not even know how to digest a tatty old paperback if it were tossed in on top of so much mess.

I am not worthy of your love: not good, nor beautiful, nor clever. I don't deserve anything, and yet I ask for you. Not for any reason except that I want a bumper bundle treat. A giant ice cream with meringue, cream and nuts, and a cherry on top of that. I want the cinema, the theatre, dinner out and a party, all in one night. I want a frilly frothy dress with sequins all over, and diamonds on top of the sequins.

So much of a super duper treat having you would be to me that, as in a fairy tale, the dustbin of my life would be turned into a golden coach.

# Pamela Pickton

BOSS

Years later she was to remember how, in those days sitting in their garden, she heard over and over again the same horrific sound.  She had never heard anybody mention hearing this and repeatedly, daily, but she did.  A shriek: a scream of a small animal she supposed, in the beak of a predator flying overhead.  It was a sound of pain and terror, she thought at the time but not a call for help.  It was the ultimate sound of utter misery and terror at a fate – destruction – where the one who cried had no hope or even thoughts of rescue.

 She would lie on a deckchair in those days, in some kind of pretence to the world (or neighbours?) or to herself, that she was having a nice time.  The deckchair, two deckchairs, sat in the garden of their house.  He would like, require, that she be seen to be having a nice time.

The screeching amazed and puzzled her for she did not remember hearing it before (and indeed has not since) and she almost hated it for its daily persistence, impinging on her world.  For how could anyone nearby bear such hopeless terror and excruciating pain, and such helplessness?

 The sound trickled on the outside of her consciousness too, like another animal whimpering for attention.  For she was half acknowledging that this sound thrown up by nature was an echo or a 'pointing out' of her state of mind: being in the hands of a predator.  The thing was, she knew nobody would believe her: her whimpering inner animal was only kidding itself there was help but, in fact, was as doomed as the one in the claws of Mr. Relentless.

If the abuse were physical it might have been easier, though what proof does any woman really have, what belief can she engage, which is not followed by, ' you must have displeased him`?  For displease him she did, by not assenting to the role of passive victim.  No, it was more than that, he had spelled it out: she was meant to be happy simply by providing him with happiness - or its appearance.

For he had once told her that he did not care what people thought of him so long as they were polite.  Mr. Empty Husk seen to be in a nice life in a nice house with a nice wife, and he was actually ecstatic with that.  It was what he had decided on and so to have it, meant he had control.  In the early days, when she had complained about something, he had told her to be quiet or he would 'show her who was boss.'  He often spoke of telling people who was Boss.

Control and power were all and that was his problem with her.  It was not that she did anything wrong, for she scurried like the victim mouse to do his bidding.  No, it was simply that she was not happy that made him tighten his grip on her.  She supposed the vicious silences were meant to deaden her spirit, make her do anything rather than endure that. Be happy, so she would not go. Be happy so he had control even of her soul.

Vicious, tangible silences and bullying - but there was more than that.  She was frightened but she did not know why.  Maybe she was frightened of the silences and bullying but, when she thought about it, she realised that she was frightened because that was what he wanted her to be.  There was something else too.  It was difficult to work out, but she knew that in those silences there was a knife coming through that was sheer punishment.  Again, she didn't know why, but supposed it was just that she was being shown what she would get if she did not toe the line – which she usually did.  It was so to fill her with terror and a sense of being wrong that she was immobilised. Sometimes she felt that he simply enjoyed having the power to make her scared.

# Pamela Pickton

So, she could not escape any more that the soft boned animal in the talon grip could escape.    Or could she?

They attended regular meetings of their Residents' Association.  She had to be seen to be at his side, smiling and well turned out, but of course she could not gainsay him in any proposals or discussion, and therefore rarely opened her mouth.  Nor could she open her mouth about her imprisonment, but could she get the message across in some other way?  At the meeting they sat in a large circle in the anteroom of the local church.  The meetings were frequent: the estate was new and there were a lot of teething problems.  There were also social events to be discussed, as well as the arrangements for gardening and cleaning.

One week, without changing her position and without, she hoped, changing her facial expression, she tried to get her pleas out through her eyes alone.  She sat staring, looking at first this one then that, but nobody caught her eye and stayed, nobody noticed. At the next meeting, she made her eyes burn into the eyes of the person directly across the room from her.    They looked away, embarrassed.

There was one member of the committee who she had always thought looked kind, and at a later meeting she found him sitting directly opposite to her.  She fixed her eyes on his, hoping that he would read in hers the desperation, the fear, the imprisonment - and the pleading.

'Are you all right?' he approached the married couple as they were leaving. 'You seemed to be trying to say something.  Were you too shy?'
'Oh I expect she was just not concentrating,' Mr. Put Down told him. 'Little bit of a flibbertigibbet, but a real chatterbox when she gets going and full of quite outrageous opinions, the complete opposite of mine.  But

# IN A PLACE OF DISCONNECTION

I hope as a husband I am the 'new man'. And she's certainly quite a modern miss, ha-ha.'

She stared at the man again next time, trying to push her soul across the room though her eyes. Oh please let him see that she was in trouble.

'Are you sure you are all right?'
He caught her alone this time because the Chairman had grabbed Mr. Pillar of the Community. She smiled and said that of course she was fine, all the while letting her eyes try to tell him something else.. All she could manage was to go on staring at the man, tongue tied, hoping he would do the impossible and know all from her eyes. The man stared back questioningly, almost equally pleadingly, as though begging her to say something, when an arm came around her.

'I want a private word with your wife,' said Mr. Kind, looking white and shocked.

'There is nothing you can need to say to my wife that you cannot say in front of me.' The man stared at her baffled and she...she changed her eyes, put on a smile.

'What did you tell that man?' he asked her when they got home. Then said the same thing a thousand different ways all night, and lived the next week pushing out spears of punishing silence.

For the next two meetings of the Residents' Association, she sat quietly with head lowered. Only once, hearing the kind man speak, she looked up and let her eyes meet his again, hoping that her eyes would say it all, tell above all that she wanted to tell, but could not. The next evening when the phone rang she picked up the receiver and said the number.
'How are you?' she recognised the voice, 'What is it, can't you tell me?'

Her husband came and took the receiver from her (she was not supposed to answer the telephone when he was in the house) and asked whom it was. The line went dead.

'Wrong number?' she suggested.

'I hope so,' he said, looking all the punishment that she knew was coming.

'I don't think you should come to the meetings anymore,' he wiped a finger across the shelf and inspected it for dust. 'You have more than enough to do here. They have far too many of those meetings in my opinion, but I am not one to shirk my duty.'

The man noticed that she was no longer there in the church hall, and he looked at the husband, recalling his tone when he had repeated his home telephone number. He wondered if the girl went out to a job and hoped the man did not work from home. He dialled her number in his lunchtime, she answered, he said who he was and there was a long silence before she hung up on him.

That silence to him was as all telling as her piercing stares. There was something the matter and the girl wanted to tell, yet was unable to. He would have to go there, in the day, and hope that alone with her he might dissolve that shell, that armour of fear, through which only her eyes broke through. He did not know what he had visions of - rescuing her, carrying her off? He was pretty sure the 'respectable husband' was a phoney, probably a bully.

He did not work far from the estate where they both lived, so he took off in his lunch hour one day. He left his car in case she were not alone and it were recognised by Mr. Miss-Nothing. For the same reason he got the taxi to drop him early, and hoped he'd find her house – on the other side to his – in those myriads of little roads, which make up a suburban estate. As he walked what seemed like a maze, his dazed thoughts followed the roads` confused pattern.All right, there was no car to recognise, but how would he disguise himself?

He was working on what reason to give for calling, if the husband happened to be at home – urgent news for a redevelopment plan he`d just heard of which needed immediate action? -  when the car hit him.The men were at work. The wives in the kitchen. The unseeing curtains would tell no tales.

It would seem that all the powers of the universe were in the thrall of Mister I-must-have-my-own-way. He had left something  at home and returned briefly to get it. There had not been time for anyone to have missed him at work.Well, the man had just stepped out into the road, hadn't he/? Not looking where he was going.

That would be the defence if he were found out, decided the driver, as he continued his journey. If not, and anyone noticed a bump on his car, well – he would say he had run over a dog.Well, again, he had hadn't he? What else could you call the cur who visited other men`s wives in their absence?

The Rescuer, on the stretcher, just had time to say, 'Help her, I think she is in danger.'  And the police were left with that mystery for a few weeks, before they finally decided to draw a blank. It was some weeks before she heard of his death.  There was no reason why her husband should tell her, and it was one of the residents who did.  She never knew the location of the accident and that he was killed on his way to rescue her.  Maybe if she had, it might have made a difference, just knowing how somebody had recognised, or indeed valued her.  That might have done something for her confidence.  For above all, that was what these few years of marriage had done to her.  Her self-esteem had been below floor level before she met him – why else had Mr. Con Man chosen her – and now it was down in hell.

# Pamela Pickton

Still though, sometimes, she felt a spark of life left; a flickering of life from an old intelligence, of creativity or even humour.  For example they went on holiday for a week.  'I like people to see us going on holiday together,' he had told her.  On the Saturday night when they returned home he said to her,

'Have we got any bananas?'

'No,' she said.

'Where would I have got them?' she nearly said, knowing he would have expected her, as well as packing for both of them the previous Friday, to have also gone out for food for their return and magically, as Mrs. Perfect Housewife, she would have been expected to know how to keep fresh any week-old fruit.  More, she would not have been allowed to pop out to a local shop to do it. No, as usual it would have meant travelling to a distant market where things were cheap.  It was part of his psychosis, she had long realised, that he wanted the upmarket image, told himself that they were affluent, and yet would not let them spend money.

That night, when she was in the bathroom alone, she nearly burst out laughing, remembering an old song, and she sang and danced it in a moment of unwatched freedom.

'Yes we have no bananas.

`Bananas we have none at all!'

Just supposing she had broken into that song and dance routine at the time! Would he have magicked a boater and cane from somewhere and joined her in dance? Was it all because she was no fun, all this trouble? Because she allowed herself to be bullied, instead of laughing at him, that she got all this abuse? So it was all her fault then, as she had always known it was.

But she began wondering what would happen if she did something like that.  If he knew she had been with friends, he would ask, 'What have you been telling your friends, have you been telling them about your bad husband?' Once, when one of his friends had not phoned for some time he said to her, 'you haven't been calling him have you, telling him that I'm not what I said?'

The days of silence – not speaking, sometimes not eating for days, usually followed any wish or plan of his that she opposed. And of course it always meant that she gave in. After a few months, on those days of long punishing silences or after a particularly bad night of constant, vicious verbal violence, she found herself looking at him and wondering, what does he think is going to happen? Why does he think I am not going to say something? After a three-day silence one Bank Holiday, they were due to meet some of his colleagues for dinner. They travelled there in silence, with her feeling numb and in shock and wondering if the people would notice. As soon as they got to the house he was all smiles and polite gush. Nobody would know he had not spoken at all that long weekend.

However, there was still that spark of life and hope in her and one of the major causes of his anger was her unhappiness. Maybe they could try Marriage Counselling, she thought, and suggested it. He refused saying that someone might see them going in there. Worse, a colleague of his might be a Relate voluntary worker. There would be no point anyway, she thought, exhausted. She tried to imagine how it would be if she were to speak to a counsellor about the bullying, the violence – or the sexual sickness.

 He would be humiliated but what then? Would he kill her? She knew that sometimes couples had some Relate sessions separately; say if they were too embarrassed to talk about a marriage problem in front of their partner. That would mean, though, that the counsellor would talk to the other partner about it on their own. She tried to think that he would be chastened and begin working on the marriage, on himself. Then, she knew it was more likely that he would come home and, if not kill, beat her.

Or just inflict more limitations, more imprisonments, and more silences.

She had a dream at this time, a real asleep dream, not a day time visitation as the screeching of the tiny animal had seemed to be. On the holiday that ended with the bananas, their car had been vandalised. They first knew of it when they could not unlock the doors. Somehow they had managed to do it after a while and she had been told to sit in the car, to test some of the controls. Then the doors had become inoperable again. Nor would the windows open. She had been trapped and sat there screaming, terrified. He looked at her and then left her alone while he walked a distance to telephone the Road Rescue Service.

Now, she began dreaming of being in the closed, shut car and woke with a soundless screaming in her throat. It was not until after a week of this that it came to her what that terror had been about. It had been that she knew, even if she had begun to show signs of going mad with claustrophobia, let alone dying from lack of air, he would never have smashed the windows of his beloved car for her.

He put her down so much in public. 'My wife has lost her pin number,' he had once announced to the whole bank. It came to her how things creep up on you - how at the beginning of a relationship a bit of teasing is welcome, seeming to be an intimate thing and part of a greater intimacy. She knew now that teasing can be the thin end of the wedge, where the thick end is putdowns or even ridicule.

She was allowed to go with him to a Christmas drink for the estate's residents. It followed days of silence, which themselves had followed her outburst that she could not buy a hundred pounds of Christmas cards and gifts and food with only twenty. As she listened to other couples`

# IN A PLACE OF DISCONNECTION

Christmas plans, plans that included children, and also saw the occasional tenderness pass between them; a tear escaped from her eye.At home of course she was chastised for causing him 'public humiliation'.

Over the Christmas period, they went to her brother and his wife for lunch and she felt the forbidden tears nearly escape as she stared at the mounds of sliced meat, the many vegetables, and most of all the roast potatoes that looked better than any she had seen for a long time. He and she rarely ate out of their home and she did all the cooking in it. She also had to buy what seemed like twenty pounds of groceries for five.

They all had second helpings of the dinner and there were two bottles of wine. At the end of the meal there were still two roast potatoes on the serving dish and a glass of wine left in the bottle.
    'Come on, who`s going to finish everything off?' Almost before finishing the question, her brother caught her wistful eye.
    'You'd like it, wouldn't you?' He put the potatoes on her plate and emptied the bottle into her glass.
    'Oh yes,' said Mr. Jovial-Teasing-Husband. 'Can't take her anywhere. Always finishes off all the food, can't get enough alcohol.'

And her fantasies about the bananas and the Relate Officer finally came to life, unchecked through her dammed up lips that could no longer hold them in.

'What do you think?' She stood up. 'Of course I soak up, suck up, any extra drink and food I can get.' She grabbed the car keys from the table and raced for the door.
    'Do you think I get enough food with you? I am forever starving. For food, for life, for love. For real sex,' she shouted the last words as she slammed the front door.

# Pamela Pickton

As she started the engine up she could hardly bear to picture his humiliation. What could he say, now that all was revealed? He would surely crumble. She did not know where she was going, but she had said it. The secret was out. Maybe now everyone would come to her rescue: realise how it had been for her (for he would surely reveal all now, would be giving himself away in that room right now, throwing one of his bizarre mental tantrums). Her brother would help her, keep him from her, and go with her every inch of the way through what she knew would be a nasty divorce.

Back in the room he coughed and wiped his lips on the table napkin.

'I must apologise to you,' he said, 'for my wife's outburst. I have not liked to tell you before, but I am afraid she is unbalanced, and is becoming increasingly so. I am glad to have it come out at last. Now I can tell you. She needs treatment, maybe more. She might...' he sighed and momentarily covered his face with his napkin. 'I am very much afraid she may have to go in somewhere.' He sat with his hands neatly folded; looking wistful, looked down at his hands and then looked up at the brother and his sister-in-law with pained eyes.

The brother jumped up and grabbed his own car keys from their hook.

'Come on,' he said. 'We can catch her up. I don't suppose she drives fast, does she?'

'No,' he said, standing up and pulling on his coat, 'she does not drive well at all. That is why I have not allowed it before. I am afraid...' He looked almost tearful, 'that she is not very competent at anything.'

'We'll pull over beside her,' her brother said as he sped off in the direction she would have had to go before meeting the main junction.

'Force her to the edge, to stop. She'll let you get in won't she? She'll let you get in the car with her?'

# IN A PLACE OF DISCONNECTION

'Oh yes,' he said, sitting bold upright, calm and controlled.
'Oh yes,
`She'll let me in the car.'

# Pamela Pickton

COMEUPPANCE

It all began when she heard a radio discussion about Capital Punishment, and something that was said made her pause. For one speaker pointed out that murder is the only crime punished in kind: for having killed, the murderer loses his life. You do not, he explained, burgle the burglar, mug the mugger, and rape the rapist. What would you do, appoint a Public Rapist?

This was a point that she had never heard before, and it set her thinking. Should anyone who has stolen, be made to pay back what was taken, or its equivalent, that would not be the same as being burgled; he would only be without what was not his in the first place. If he were sentenced to give back double, or even more, he would sustain loss, as his victim had done, but that still would not be the same. There would be none of the terror of sudden attack, or any of the outrage, the feelings of invasion and defilement, which are experienced by those who come home to find their house ransacked. One of the worst parts of having been attacked, or of having anything taken from you, is the element of surprise and shock; and if a perpetrator knows his sentence, he never experiences that.

There was no way her destroyer could be punished in kind. How could he be condemned to find himself married to somebody who slowly revealed himself as a monster? There would be none of the shock she had experienced, for he would be forewarned. She had been caught in the blissful hope of new beginnings with her defences down, and there was no way to replicate that slow and gradual revelation which had been hers after marriage; that realisation that she had not known what he was. That creeping up of awareness that it was only going to get worse.

Not only could he not be made to suffer, but what he had inflicted he might do it again. This was her fear, but she was still in touch with one of their neighbours and she constantly begged her to warn any new woman he got his clutches on. For, with all the charm of the deceiver, he would easily snare someone else. Yet although part of her did not want him to marry again, to destroy someone else, another part of her hoped he would marry and meet his match.

The only revenge for a man like that would be for somebody to pull the wool over his eyes, be cruel once they were married, then when he could stand no more, do him out of the house, the money, everything.

Yes, that was what she wanted to happen to him.

Of course that would have to be a very different woman from herself. Meekness, gentleness and above all self doubting, those were the qualities he looked for in a woman and that is exactly what she had provided.

Self-doubt was the chief requirement. For to an extent she had believed she had to do what he wanted, had never believed that her own needs or rights were as important as those of others. She had been an innocent, unsuspecting soul and her good nature had for a long time prevented her from believing what she saw with her own eyes, until it was too late. He could not mean it; she had persuaded herself at first, and resolved to 'work on' the marriage.

One thing she knew for certain was that he would never allow himself to become tied to a woman who was not low in expectations, unassuming, and with his preferred dash of guilt thrown in. When, as they frequently did, people told her to put it all behind her, 'get on with her life' as they put it, she told them that she could not until certain needs had been met. People who have been through any kind of atrocity require something akin to the old 'Rites of Passage'. As coming through bereavement involves passing through various stages, so she needed certain processes for healing to take place.

Anyway, how was she supposed to get on with her life, right at the bottom of life's ladder and totally winded as she was?

He had conned her into marriage, got her to sell her flat and move into his with the promise that they would pool assets and buy a bigger place between them. Then, on all kinds of pretexts, he had dipped into her savings account, so they did not move and by the time she fled she had nothing. His flat? Well, that had been his all along, hadn't it?

There had been all sorts of reasons to run through her money, first refurbishing his flat. 'I want everything to be perfect for my bride' and 'it will help us to sell it, darling.' A new car, safer, so that she would be protected. In a similar way he excused his job change which had run away with the greatest amount of the equity from her flat. It was to be for their mutual benefit one day, but meanwhile he needed expensive career counselling and then a period of retraining.

Sometimes she wondered if it had all been part of some carefully worked out plan, to render her penniless and therefore tied to him and his cruelty. A pre-marriage contract you could almost say, but one made by himself to himself. In the end she decided that the only way for her to get on with her life - to heal - was first of all to remove herself from the locality. As she only had a rented place now it was easy. As to her work, well that was the unskilled sort that her nervous state dictated, and that kind of job was available anywhere. She told friends that they would not be able to contact her, because she could be anywhere but that she would call them when she was more in control of things.

'I am going to work on myself,' she told them.

When, after many months, she decided to get in touch with her old area, she learned that he had indeed found a replacement for her. However, there was no point in her pleas to warn the girl off. That had already been done, but she would hear nothing against him. Naturally his ex was eager to hear all about this new bride-to-be, for she was that already, and particularly how this bride compared with herself.

His fiancée was meek and gentle, she was told. Well, so had she been: that was the kind of woman he sought.

# IN A PLACE OF DISCONNECTION

She was surprised to hear that in appearances the girl was nothing like her. Her amazement was obviously clear and she explained it by saying that men usually go for the same type. Well, she was told, their heights were probably the same, but it was an average height after all. Her face might be similarly small and round, but her features were so different that overall there was no likeness. The face was rather doll like with the small upturned nose and high cheekbones.

Yes, she did rather resemble a plastic doll, they agreed. Just what he would want, surely - a puppet? But what made her seem so different from her predecessor, however, were her clothes and general style. She wore short, pleated skirts and tiny heels and her hair was mousy and cut in a bob. 'Old fashioned' was how she heard the girl described and nothing like her with her somewhat arty clothes and long, highlighted hair that she always wore tied back or piled on top. Yes, in spite of being married to a man who really wanted a plastic doll, an old fashioned wife aproned in old fashioned obedience, she had retained her bohemian appearance and throughout the whole episode wondered why he had taken on someone like her.

For he was Establishment Man - traditional in appearance and custom. On the other hand, she supposed, marrying her had appealed to his desire to appear normal, open minded, all embracing. After all, most people nowadays are letting their hair down a bit. To be seen with a slightly whacky wife presented a desired image.

Therefore she was not at all surprised to hear that in some ways the girl was that, for not only was the marriage ceremony to take place in one of the new authorised venues, but the bride had announced she was writing the service herself. Their mutual friend was amazed that he was allowing it but she herself understood; especially when informed that the girl`s reason was that she liked words and wrote a bit of poetry.

# Pamela Pickton

As his ex she knew him better than the neighbour and explained that he would love this. It was the same as putting up with her mildly unorthodox appearance, serving to reinforce him as the generous husband. And no doubt he found dabbling in a bit of poetry rather amusing and on the same lines as doing embroidery. When she voiced her belief that the marriage would not go through she was asked why she did not turn up on the day, sit at the back and slip out before he saw her.

But she did not want her face to be seen at that wedding.

It was some time before she was able to make another call to her informer and when she did an excited shriek of gossip about to spill forth met her ear. The wedding service had been quite a turn up for the books, and the work of our gentle poetess not quite the flowery nonsense imagined. Skilfully, in fact, she had written the words and vows of the ceremony in such a way that the creeping up to the coup d'état at the end was almost imperceptible.

The bride's vows had been simple: just that she would always have her husband's deepest desires at heart. His words however, written by the bride, were other and oh so cleverly worded. As a traditional husband he would indeed expect obedience, but in return he would be the old-fashioned provider and protector. These vows then led quite naturally to what at the end amounted to a marriage contract. The Registrar read out the words she had written and the bridegroom repeated them. It had been clever the way those vows led to an acknowledgment that in making marriage vows he was under obligation to keep them and would be answerable to that congregation if he did not. The 'contract' followed easily from that.

As an honourable man he would look after his wife in marriage and, God forbid, beyond. Should the marriage end, she would be housed and maintained.

The neighbour described how he had just stood there, looking frozen, and whispered the words he had to repeat, squared his shoulders and lifted his chin.

# IN A PLACE OF DISCONNECTION

'I thought, I would have thought, he would crumple,' the ex-wife said.

For indeed if told that this was to happen, she would have guessed that. Or that he would refuse, really blow and reveal his true self.

Or that he would get out of it in some cunning way.

He might have said that he had come to the service not really wanting to go through with it and until this moment had been plucking up courage to speak - that he was still in love with his ex, that he did not have enough to offer, that he fully agreed with the vows and the 'contract,' but felt she deserved a stronger man and a better provider. Anything.

'But from what you told me,' said her informant, 'he's wily – he'll be up to something: he'll get out of it, think of something.'

'Yes,' she agreed. 'Appearances are all too him and that includes seeming decency as well as status. But what he is probably thinking now is that the contract will never hold water, never be counted legally binding. He thinks he will find a way out, if anything ever goes wrong between them.'

Wrong for him it was.

He could hardly understand what was happening, or even that it was happening. She had been so docile. The first thing was when she had said she was too unwell to get out of bed to get his early morning cup of tea; worse she had made him get some tea for her. With the other, if she ever complained of being unwell, even once asking him get the shopping for her, he had always squashed it by saying that he felt ill too. 'I can`t help you, darling, I don`t feel well myself.' Acting unwell is an easy one: who can disprove it?

This little bitch had got under his defences reminding him of his boasting to people how he was a New Man and how he loved his little wifey. She didn't threaten to tell people if he neglected her, oh no, it was far more subtle than that.

# Pamela Pickton

'Won't you feel wonderful, darling, when I tell all our friends how you got me tea in bed?'

It was a slow imperceptible creeping away from the obedient, serving wife, through cunning tactics which still held all the old winsomeness, 'til now she filled his life with horror. Somehow she had known what to do. Like reminding him what a fine upstanding man he was and how the old school establishment man puts his woman on a pedestal.

If he reprimanded her on the spending of money - which the other one would never have dared to do - she reminded him that appearances were all and that he would not want his wife to be seen out in rags, or not able to have lunches out like her friends. All his life he had got people to do what he wanted and most people were easy to intimidate. But he recalled how his mother had snapped orders at him and he had been too frightened of her to disobey. Most people had never dared. If they did he was lost – as though his mother were there again.

When they first met and married, she had been working full time but now she gave up her job and took a part-time one, mornings only. Now, she was not only eating up all his salary, but was fast depleting his savings too. His murmurings that they could not really manage brought the sharp reminder that he had told everyone he wanted the best for her and that no wife of his worked. In softer tones, she stroked his hand and said that all she ever wanted was to be there with his meal when he came home.

'And we do have your savings, darling.'

When he pointed out that those were fast vanishing, she smiled sweetly and said, 'Oh come on. What are you worrying about? You have a lot more money than you are letting on. You told me that you have a secret account, saved on the back of your last wife.'

When had he told her that?

At first he thought he would do something. Nobody got the better of him and that wretched contract would never stand up in court. But somehow he became weary as time went on. The stuffing seemed to have been knocked out of him. The cruelties were only little ones, but lots of little mice nibbling at you constantly, probably amounts to the same pain in the end as one big bite from a lion or a shark.

Sometimes she was not in when he got home: once even when she had taken his key to give to a tradesman, so he was locked out. Once or twice she cooked a spaghetti meal when he had told her at the outset that he loathed any form of pasta.

'But darling, I love it. Am I never to have what I like? Oh, shall I go out for a pasta, sweetie; have spaghetti for lunch once a week? There's that new Italian restaurant. Some of the girls go to it. A bit expensive for us perhaps, but...'

In shops and restaurants, in front of sales girls or friends, she always chose the most expensive thing, smiling as he signed the credit slip and telling everyone how he gave her everything she wanted.

She got up early at weekends, when he was tired from a week's work, and he was woken by the noise of the vacuum cleaner, outside the bedroom door or even inside it.

'I wanted to finish early, darling,' she explained, 'so that we can have the day together.'

In bed she read 'til the small hours, the light causing him to wake and sleep fitfully.

He was tired and he began to look ill. Then came the bombshell. One day she looked at him and said that she could see he was not happy and thought they should end things. When he objected and whimpered about the contract and that he would be ruined, she replied that was his problem. She could not live with such a miserable man.

He blustered and tried calling her darling and, saying how much he loved her, even pleading that they work on it. She cut him short. She wanted to end it she told him, looking fierce.

He repeated that he faced financial ruin.

# Pamela Pickton

'Win some, lose some,' she smiled.

The ex called her friend and said she was back in town. Could they meet soon?

'She's left him,' said the neighbour on the phone.

'Have you heard? He looks dreadful. Apparently she's blown most of his money. He'll have to re-mortgage to house her, and if she gets awarded maintenance he does not know how he will live.'

As she walked up to the table in the pub, her friend looked surprised to see her, went back to watching the door, but she sat down anyway.

'Oh,' said the neighbour, 'what are you doing here? I thought you'd just run away from him. I'm waiting for ...for his first ex,'

Then she spoke, and watched realisation dawn on the neighbour's face. It felt good to be using her voice again

'It was you all the time?'

'I had a nose job, cheekbones... the lot.'

And she explained how she had wanted him to know what it was like: to find yourself married to someone who changed overnight after the wedding, then became bullying and cruel - spent your money, ran roughshod over your life.

When it was pointed out to her that the marriage would not be valid, that she would get nothing out of it, she confessed that she had never meant it to go this far. She had expected it to end at that marriage service. She had fully expected that, and she had just wanted him to have the shock of being duped, perhaps behave in a way that revealed what he was really like, reveal the nasty self he kept hidden from public view. She thought that he would explode with anger, but that what would come through was that he was basically selfish and mean.

'So it's over. You have had your revenge. What now? `

'I could go on living with him.'

# IN A PLACE OF DISCONNECTION

'Why don't you come clean? Have another go at it. After all he sounds as though he is completely different now.'

'No he isn't! He wouldn't !

`You don't understand, with a man like that it is either him or you! It is all about power. He can only operate in power relationships. Either he bullies or you do. There is no equal, no level meeting: you are either up on the seesaw or down on the ground. I think it all began with his mother. She bossed him. So when he got a wife he bossed her. Even I did it once in the first marriage. Once he was doing something that was making my teeth grate and for an instant I forgot my usual fear and told him to stop it: to shut up.'

'And he took it?'

'Of course! Which is why he has "taken" this second marriage.'

'But you've made your point now. You don't want to go back. He's had punishment enough.'

'Has he?' she said.


At first he was pleased at the reconciliation. She was fairly sweet for a while and at least he would not have to go through the public disgrace of yet another divorce so soon after the last one.

She did not mean to go on behaving badly, at least no more so than before. But one cold wet Saturday she decided to go out for the day, to a new Gallery that was opening in town and blow the weekly shop.

She looked in the fridge and saw there was very little food in it, only a couple of eggs and the end of a loaf. And, deciding that she needed a good breakfast before a day out, she made herself scrambled eggs on toast. There was not enough for him and he sat snivelling with some cold coming on or something, and complaining that there was no food in the house.

'You don`t want me buying lunches out, darling, not on your pathetic pay. This way I`ll only need a snack midday. You can get out to the shops, can't you?'

# Pamela Pickton

And she left him with the scrambled egg pan to wash up.

When she got home he looked worse: coughing and wrapped in a blanket. He had not been able to get out for food. She had brought herself in fish and chips.

'I thought you would have eaten,' she said and proceeded to eat half the rather large portion and then scrape what was left into the bin.

By the time she had tidied up from her day, admiring her knick-knacks from the Gallery shop, she found him in the living room watching television, still huddled in his blanket.

'What rubbish are you watching?' she remarked, going over to the television and changing the channel.

He went to bed and for a moment she was shocked at what she had done. She was just playing games wasn't she? Just wanting him to get what she had got? To experience the kind of misery she had felt. Like when he 'lost' the letter that told her she had won a competition. Just snatched up special chocolates given to her by a grateful boss and given them, instead of wine, when they went for dinner with friends. When he continued to give her details of torture he had read of, although she begged him to stop.

He lay in bed shivering. As she got in beside him, she thought that maybe he really did have the flu, as he'd said, and not just a cold as she had jeered at him it was. His continuous cough was keeping her awake. She lay there for some time then got out of bed.

The sound of wind and rain made her look out of the window. It was open a chink, but then they needed fresh air, with his germs. Still, it was very cold. If she were going to take a sleeping bag to the sofa, she would need an extra blanket. She would have to take one off him. He was asleep, he wouldn`t notice and serve him right for keeping her awake. He wouldn`t come after her. He was too weak to get out of bed.

# IN A PLACE OF DISCONNECTION

As she went to go out of the door, she looked back at him and gave a little smile…
And opened the window wider.

Just a little bit.

# Pamela Pickton

THE WATCHING EYE

'She would not have been able to do that if a gnome had been watching her with his vigilant eye.'

(Margaret Yorke: Intimate Kill)

I must tidy up. It will be all right if I can just tidy up the mess. I mustn't let Mummy see what I've done.

I have always made sure I tided up, cleaned up, after that first time. It was when I wet my knickers. I was about three, I think, and Mummy was so cross. She took the knickers off me, and held them, kind of stretched out by her two hands in front of me. They were all sort of steaming. I know now of course that wee is hot. Mummy kept saying how naughty I was, how bad and what a dirty, dirty girl I was.

She wrapped the knickers in newspaper and put the lot on the kitchen boiler, where she burnt rubbish. Then she took off all my clothes and threw them into the big thing called a copper that she did the washing in. She said that some of them needed hand washing and might shrink in the boiler, but she said better that than that they be 'contaminated.' I did not know what that long word meant but I have always remembered it. Mummy used the word quite a lot. She said it when she made Daddy take his muddy boots off before coming into the kitchen, and when she nagged him to scrub his hands after any sort of a job.

When I was a bit older, I came home from a friend's house one day and asked her why my friend's parents slept in the same bedroom but she and Daddy did not. I had thought it was because they had lots of children. We only had me. Though as time went by, I came to notice that my friend's house was very big and that they had a 'spare' room.

Mummy used the word contaminate then.

# IN A PLACE OF DISCONNECTION

Later still, when we learnt about babies at school, I asked Mummy why I had never seen her and Daddy kiss. She used the word then as well.

She never let me have a pet animal. I don't have to tell you the word she used.

So, after taking all my clothes off on that wet knicker day, she put me into the big stone sink and filled it with very hot water. Then she scrubbed me with the big brush she normally used to scrub the floor. She made me stand up in the sink, and I bumped my legs on the taps, and she scrubbed and scrubbed my bottom still it stung. Then, when it was already stinging, she slapped it `til I thought she would never stop and I could not bear it.

So I always clear up. Never let her know what I've done. I was a lot older when I next wet my knickers, too old to be doing it. But I had been out at a friend's house playing and had not liked to ask to go. On the way home I did it. There was only an alley between our two houses and nobody saw. I took the wet things off and threw them into a bush, then ran back home hugging my skirt around me. Mummy was busy scrubbing the floor so I said I had come to get my skipping rope. But as well as the skipping rope I took my pocket money out of its secret place. I didn`t know whether Mummy would find out or how I would replace the money in case she did, but that was a problem for another day. I walked as far as the village and found the shop where I had seen Mummy buy things like socks and knickers, there were plenty of pairs just like the ones I wore. I paid for them and put them on in the public lavatories where I had also been with Mummy. I threw the paper bag in a bin.

I could always say that one of my friends had stolen the money, couldn't I?

# Pamela Pickton

It is always all right just so long as I clear up. That's what I've learned. Not to get told off, that's the only thing. Like that time at school and the teacher's cup. The teacher on playground duty had taken her mug of tea out onto the playground, I suppose because it was such a freezing cold day. When she had finished drinking, I was nearest to her and she asked me to take the cup into the teachers' room. Round the corner, out of sight, I slipped on some ice and the mug broke. I was scared. What would the teacher say? What would the school do? Worst of all, would they tell Mummy? I had a big hanky in my pocket because I had caught what Mummy called a bit of a chill with the snowy weather, so I scraped up the broken bits and wrapped them in the hanky. I cut my hand a bit. Then, I ran round to the back of the building to where I knew the big bins stood and threw it all in there. I told Mummy I had thrown the hanky away because it was so snotty and I thought it would contaminate her washing. (Oh I was getting so clever, don't you see?). She noticed the cuts on my hand and I said I had got them falling over on some ice, which was not completely a lie was it?

Everything is always all right as long as you clear up. Once, Mummy let me have my tea in the front room because she was busy scouring and scrubbing the kitchen. It was called Spring Cleaning I think, but anyway it was not finished when I came home from school. So I was allowed as a special treat to sit in the best room with a tray on my lap and watch the television which I was rarely allowed to do, and I dropped my plate of cake onto the floor, onto the best carpet. The plate did not break, because of the carpet, but there were crumbs and lumps of cake all over. Although I picked it all up, and ate it all up quickly before I had any more accidents, there were still so many bits that were too big to pick up, however hard I tried. So I got down on my hands and knees and licked them up. It was horrible and I got fluffy bits in my mouth along with the crumbs, but - just so long as Mummy did not find out....

# IN A PLACE OF DISCONNECTION

It won't matter, I repeat to myself, just so long as nobody finds out, nobody sees - as long as Mummy does not see. It can be as if it had never happened.

I had had another accident with knickers when I was a bit older. When I took them off one night, I saw some red spots in them. I didn't know what they were but I knew it must be in some way dirty. I didn't want Mummy to see. She always inspected the washing, particularly the underwear, before it went into the copper to be boiled. So that evening I sneaked them into the bath with me and washed them in the bath water. Then I sneaked back into my bedroom and hung them out of the window to dry, hidden behind the curtain. In the morning, they were fit enough to put in Mummy`s washing basket.

Once, when I had dropped ink on one of the pages of my school exercise book, I tore it out. When Teacher noticed a page missing, I told her that a visiting baby cousin had ripped it.

It won't matter as long as I can clear up I think now, beginning to see the full extent of what I have done and just what I have to 'tidy away.'

Those red spots came back in my pants again, and in the end Mummy had found out and had told me what it was.
'It happens to the best of us,' Mummy had said, but I had known it was a dirty thing all along. Although I had been told that what was called 'The Curse' came every month, every month I had hoped it wouldn't, hoped it would  'go away`.

Then, a few years later, the worst thing of all that I had had to clear up. I had done the bad thing, the contaminating thing. I had let a boy kiss me. We both went to the church youth club and carried on kissing long after we had both left school.  I had always scrubbed my

# Pamela Pickton

mouth with the horrible soap and the cold water of the church hall before I went home. I liked kissing but I knew I mustn't let Mummy know. Mummy was always busy spring cleaning or scouring. All she said when I asked her about growing up and getting married, was that I must just work hard at my job in the department store and try to better myself, whatever that meant. The boy had wanted to do more than kiss and I let him. I found I liked it and wondered why it was called contaminating. Then I found out. So that is why kissing is contaminating, I thought, when I took myself alone to a doctor and found I was pregnant.

The terror: What would Mummy do? What would Mummy say? I could hardly bear to think of her face and imagine the humiliation as when the wet knickers had been dangled before me. Like rubbing my nose in it.

Nothing mattered except that Mummy should never find out, and scarcely knowing what to do or how to do it, I found I had taken a bus to a distant town and an unknown doctor.

` I must clear it up,' I said to him, 'I must clear up this mess. I always have to tidy up my messes so that Mummy will not find out. She'll say I am contaminated.'

He was looking at me strangely as I said all this, but he looked a kindly man.

'Look,' he said, 'it is not legal to end a pregnancy, but I can see you are distressed, so there is something I could do.'

Later he told me he was to confess to his wife (though he dare not to a colleague) that he had felt forced `to help the girl`.

'She looked mad. I don`t know much about her, but I tell you she`s not normal. I had to do it - didn't I? Tell me I was right to give her those pills.'

Telling me like that – I think now I must have driven him a bit mad too.

# IN A PLACE OF DISCONNECTION

I took the pills, without Mummy knowing of course. It took weeks but then one night I woke with cramping pains. I got out of bed to walk around with the pain, just as I had found it helped a bit with period pains. And then clots of blood started falling on the floor. Fortunately, I didn't wear underwear beneath my nightdress or I would have had dirty knickers again. In the depth of night I crept downstairs and found the pile of newspapers kept by the boiler. I took them to my bedroom and wrapped up the blood and the mess. I knew mother slept soundly - with all that scrubbing you would - and Dad...well,it seemed all Dad ever did was being at work or working in the garden, or asleep. He found it hard enough to wake in the mornings. So I went to the bathroom and washed out the nightie and hung it in the airing cupboard. It would be dry before mother noticed in the morning. If she asked, I would say I got dressed early for work because I had to be in early. Finally, I got the toilet cleaning cloth from the bathroom and washed my bedroom floor; linoleum not carpet, so I did not have to lick up the last bits like the crumbs. I threw the cloth on the boiler and would just deny all knowledge of it. I knew where the clean ones were in the kitchen drawer and I hoped that Mummy didn't count them any more than the teachers had counted the cups.

Then, I went back to bed, shivering with no nightie, and had to get up early to put the nightie back on my bed and appear to leave early for work, when really I would be walking the cold streets. Years later, when I told someone, they had asked me how I could possibly have had an abortion under my mother's roof without her knowing about it.

'She was asleep,' I explained.

'But you did not call for her?'

'I didn't tell Mummy anything,` I tried to explain, `I had to clear up my mess. Make it as though it had never happened. She would have said I was contaminated.'

# Pamela Pickton

So you see I must clear up now. What I see in front of me is just another something to clear up, so that Mummy will not see.

Nobody must find out.

I hear someone snivelling, whimpering, in the distance. It is as though all those other younger selves were crying, as they never cried - at the dirty knickers, at the broken cup and the cake crumbs. At those blobs on the lino, that might have been a baby.

This part of me has always been thinking, mustn`t let Mummy see, mustn`t let Mummy see - got to clear up. Nobody must see.

Far away comes the sobbing as though it were coming from somebody else.

Is there anybody else?

What am I going to do? I get hold of the broom but I can't sweep this up like the spilled crumbs or broken bits of cup. No, like the teacher's cup I have to wrap the mess up, but not in a hanky. That`s what I must do. I get a dustbin bag but that does not cover it all, so I get another one, one at each end. It is not easy to pull the bags over, right down. Somehow it reminds me of trying to put a duvet cover on and I hear mad laughter in the distance. But I wont be able to carry it like this. Covered or not, it is too heavy, not like the cup. That had been easy and the school had never found the broken bits in the bin. If only I can hide this, hide what I've done, nobody will ever find out.

If nobody saw, nobody would know. Just so long as nobody was watching.

But I can't carry a big bag like that. I could carry lots of little bags, one by one. If it were in bits.

# IN A PLACE OF DISCONNECTION

A knife. I am holding a knife. That is no good. It doesn't work. I run down to the garden shed, get the axe, the saw - an electric saw.

Mummy has a gardener now. Everything would be sharp, be in working order. When had Daddy gone? I couldn't remember Daddy going. Was he dead or just gone away? He had always seemed a bit of a shadow really, not really there. It had only been Mummy.

Perhaps he was not dead at all. Oh, Daddy, Daddy.
The sobbing grows louder in the distance as I chop and hack and saw.

A girl friend once told me that she always felt her mother there, long after she had married and no longer lived with her mother, and even when her mother was dead. 'If I don't clean the house one week, or if I leave the washing in the machine all day, I can feel her looking over my shoulder, disapproving,' she said.

I had not got married. So long, oh so long, it seems to have been just me and Mummy, with Mummy telling me I was no good and why did I not get promotion at the Department Store? And, of course, that I would never get married - who would want me?

In the end I got so tired of being told I didn't deserve anything and shouldn't even want anything. I did not mean to do it.
'Oh Mummy I didn't mean it and I know I am a bad girl.'
The tears are running through my nose now.
I chop and hack.
Must tidy up. Must tidy up.
I saw and saw.
Must hide the mess. Must hide the mess.
I pile the bits into bags.
It's all right, it's all going to be all right.
I sweep the last pieces into the last bag.

# Pamela Pickton

If only I could just clear up, it would all go away! Be as though it had never happened. I run out and get the barrow. It reminds me of a doll`s pram. Mummy would not let me have a doll's pram, or a doll. I never had a baby either.

Dragging the barrow into the kitchen, I begin to heap it full of the plastic bags. And it feels like a river of tears - starting from a long way away, from a long time ago – are pouring down my cheeks, filling my mouth, splashing onto the floor
Maybe they'll wash the blood. Maybe they'll wash the blood.
Oh don't let me have to lick it up.
I drag the barrow down to the compost heap and begin shovelling the compost to one side. That makes a kind of dip in the pile, so If I put it in there and cover it with the compost....
Soon be cleared up, soon be all right.
Just so long as nobody sees...

...But I had forgotten the gnome.

The garden gnome stands just a few yards from me and he is looking at me. It seems he is looking right at me with his eye.
Somebody has seen.
I fall to my knees blowing my nose on my dress. The gnome was watching.

I crawl on my hands and knees the two miles to the Police Station. I don't know whether it is blood or tears or snot gurgling into my mouth. My hands and knees are hurting and getting bloody. But they were probably bloody anyway.

I cut my hands on the broken cup and told Mummy it was the frosty ground. Could I tell the policeman that the blood now was just from crawling? It feels like all the

186

# IN A PLACE OF DISCONNECTION

people of the world are sobbing through me, and as if all my hidden secrets were found out.


On the steps of the Police Station she finally fell flat.
They found her curled into a ball and whimpering.
'I never had a doll and I never had a baby. Mummy wouldn't let me. She made me go to work and stay with her and all we ever did was clean and scour and stop ourselves becoming contaminated. I thought I was clearing up so Mummy wouldn't see.'

What had been the point of clearing up?
Mummy had seen it all.
It was Mummy she was clearing up.
Mummy she had chopped up.
Mummy she had killed.

# Pamela Pickton

DIARY ENTRIES OF PAIN, COLLECTED FROM OCT
93' – FEB 94'

Radio talk:    'The children from Somalia arrive with
nothing, just what they have on.  They sleep anywhere at
first, perhaps on someone's floor…'
My daughter and I left our house with carrier bags.  We
slept anywhere - friends, relations.


We had been invaded by an aggressor who rode rough
shod over me, my money, my house, and my family.
Who laid waste my property, pillaged my assets, caused
devastation to my family life, my working life. Verbally and
visually raped my daughter and her friends, and left us in
this ruin.   Terrorised and tyrannised and took away my
freedom.  Made my daughter and me refugees - drove us
into exile and finally lost for us forever our homeland.
This was England
Divorce, not war.
No Aid came….

……………………………………………...........................

A Rabbi on the radio programme THOUGHT FOR THE
DAY:
'Sometimes people say, 'Oh come on, Hitler was not that
bad!'
`He wasn't…
`He was worse!'
Too right, I know the feeling.

…………………………………………………………………

Imagine you have time-travelled and you need to tell
people of some past or future horror.
And all the bright faces are around you, lights and zigzag
movements, and colours.
And no one can hear you.  They can't even see you.

…………………………………………………………………

# IN A PLACE OF DISCONNECTION

Imagine you have lived in a place of isolation: no colour, so you don't know all sorts of things exist.   You don't know any different.

And then you go to a world where all is different.   Things you did not know of.   They do not know your world exists either.   And you can't explain it to them.

.............................................................

You are down a pothole.   You fall deeper.   You have forgotten what sunshine is.   Or even human voices.   Then you hear voices above.   And fun.   But they don't know you're there.   And you can't make them hear you.

.............................................................

You are limping.   You don't know any other way than limping and pain.   But you pretend you are not, and try to keep up.   Look like other people.

.............................................................

A sob is just a sob away.
A sob away is wailing, screeching, growling.

.............................................................

Is there one friend who will come and hear me?
I am in the depths of despair.   Will one friend be the one friend I have never had?
Is there anybody who will come and listen – sympathise and comfort?   Loneliness in despair is unbearable.

.............................................................

I feel like I have come into a party in bandages.
Covered in blood –
and nobody notices.

.............................................................

I feel as if I was hit by a car, and for the last three years have been hurtling through the air.   Now that I have finally landed, I can take stock of the damage.   What was that all about?   What hit me?

.............................................................

At the Night Class overheard conversation:
'You've been on holiday, haven't you?'
'Had a good summer?'
'The last time I saw you it was bright summer.'

# Pamela Pickton

Like they say when you stop banging your head on the wall – I realised how bad it was, the hell I'd been in.  Like in a bubble all on my own.
You come from the holiday –
I come from the holocaust.

................................................................

'To be indifferent is cruelty.' ( from a book).
'Not to allow someone to express their feelings, their misery, is cruelty.' ( from the radio).

................................................................

Before this recent debacle I felt my life was like this: crawl along on your hands and knees, struggle up only to get knocked down again.  Crawl along, get up, and get knocked down again.  A big boot down from out of the sky.  Or, climb a mountain and get to the top, only to find another mountain.  Once I was with him the knocks speeded up – bang, bang and bang on the head.
Once the destruction was total, when I finally left the situation and tried to pick my life up, it was like a little metal hammer, fast, continuous, rap-rap-rap on the head.
Finally I was on the floor.
But not enough – flayed alive now.
I am this red open wound, this red raw meat,
And still people stick their knives in that.

................................................................

A man who disguised himself as a meter reader (for meter reader read lover) conned his way into my house to get my diamonds.
No, he did not run off with my diamonds.  But that was never the intention.  At least I don't think so.  I think it was for him to sit with my diamonds round his neck while I had a rope halter of power and control around mine.  To sit with the diamonds round his neck while I, with a ball and chain of fear round my feet, swept the crumbs around his.
True, he ended up without the diamonds because I took off the halter and the chains.  Though I think he may have got away with one: maybe is one diamond better off than before.

# IN A PLACE OF DISCONNECTION

But he has not been recognised as the deceiving meter reader: no prison, no fine, no pointed finger, certainly no loss.
And he has lost for me forever my diamonds. Turned them to this heap of old bricks.
Turned them to tears.

.........................................................................

I feel that I have been mugged.

.........................................................................

I feel that I have been standing at the roadside with my begging bowl.
And people are just spitting in it.

.........................................................................

'Got a job yet?' 'Are you working?' 'When are you going to get a job?'
I need a holiday not a job.
I need hospitalisation first, convalescence.
I need a stretcher not a job.

.........................................................................

I feel like the victim of a hit and run case.

.........................................................................

I feel like a bomb landed in my lovely house: my lovely home, my lovely family – my life's work. Dusted himself down, picked up his briefcase and strutted off untouched.
I feel like a big bird picked me up out of the loved house, flew round with me in its beak, and then just dropped me anywhere. This is not my house. It is just anywhere. I did not choose it. It chose me because it was all I could get.

.........................................................................

'You have choice' someone said to me, 'you can go.'
What choice? I went from one horror story to the next.

.........................................................................

Eighteen months of battering. Then two years of battering by the legal services, by everyone.

.........................................................................

'You go,' someone encouraged me. So many encouraged. Then came desertion, betrayal, hostility and punishment.

...............................................................

You know those films where she goes to the doctor and finds him in league with the devil, to the psychiatrist and finds him a traitor too? Finally, she goes to the priest, the final sanctuary, and finds him in league with the devil. So it was – the Doctor, the Law and the Church - all on the side of the man. And, since, even the Counsellor has deserted me.

...............................................................

'The sharing of pain is the beginning of healing.' (Heard on the radio)

...............................................................

I feel like Jesus on the cross, with all the disciples run away.

...............................................................

What people have done for me is like the flowers you bring someone in hospital, having  refused them operation that would have saved their life.

...............................................................

Angela (who suffered physical abuse in marriage)
'Sometimes I felt God himself had left me.'
Angela 'I feel as if I have been raped of life.'

...............................................................

'You're lucky you're not in a Refuge,' says my solicitor.
What are abused wives doing in refuges?
Why is the man not in jail?
If you assault someone in public, you are charged.
Domestic violence is unseen. Committed by the most cowardly human beings of all. Know how you might put a glass tumbler over a spider – so I feel about my experience. As Angela says not even God sees or knows. The behaviour I saw, if displayed in the work or social scene, would bring dismissal, ostracisation, even possible imprisonment. Yet because it is between the marital walls – no witness, no proof.

Why is my word not good enough?

...............................................................

# IN A PLACE OF DISCONNECTION

I feel like somebody broke into my house to rob me, and when caught said that I had dragged him in, beaten him up, planted my goods on him. And now I am in prison for that.

......................................................................

When I was with him I was trapped.  But there were doors - there was a way out.
He drove me out, through the door that led to the cell with no doors.  No way out.

......................................................................

From the film 'Pacific Heights' - On the law protecting any kind of squatter:  '...A law to protect any cretin, who moves into your property, gradually makes you bankrupt, and drives you insane.'

......................................................................

'You are so brave to have run,' they say.
Wouldn't you run if you were impaled on railings?
Painful.  Bleeding.
You know that to run means to pull yourself off, like taking a sword out of a wound. That will kill you.  But just to get away from that pain for a moment.  Not to let him have his cruel delight in watching your pain.
And the tiny hope that maybe you will heal.

......................................................................

I feel like the dreams where you are trying to scream and nothing comes out.
I feel like a leper: outside the city wall.
Nobody hears or cares or sympathises or comforts or helps.
I feel outside the Universe.
If there is any God, he can't see me
I am alone.

......................................................................

I feel like in that film WHATEVER HAPPENED TO BABY JANE.  I am lying on the beach, dying. And someone has

gone  to get me an ice- cream.

......................................................................

# Pamela Pickton

I feel so loathsome. That people left me like this, I must be so loathsome. My face must be so loathsome. I must hide it from the world. I must be so loathsome. I must take myself away from the world.

...................................................................

When people go on at me about finding work, it comes back to me, the horror of a film I once saw.
Someone was in prison, a Prisoner of War camp. She was dying, or certainly would very soon, with tuberculosis.

She had dark circles under her eyes. They come and take her out of her sick bed, out of her cell, and somehow make her walk.
Out into the sunshine.
To face the firing squad.

.

# IN A PLACE OF DISCONNECTION

Printed in the United Kingdom by
Lightning Source UK Ltd., Milton Keynes
141544UK00001B/13/P